B. M. Henz · T. Zuberbier · J. Grabbe · E. Monroe (Eds.): URTICARIA

Springer
Berlin
Heidelberg
New York
Barcelona
Budapest
Hong-Kong
London
Milan
Paris
Santa Clara
Singapore
Tokyo

B. M. Henz · T. Zuberbier · J. Grabbe · E. Monroe (Eds.)

URTICARIA

Clinical, Diagnostic and Therapeutic Aspects

With 39 Figures and 42 Tables

Springer

Prof. Dr. med. BEATE M. HENZ
Charité-Virchow Klinikum,
Medizinische Fakultät der Humboldt-Universität zu Berlin
Dermatologische Universitätsklinik und Poliklinik
Augustenburger Platz 1, D-13353 Berlin, Germany

Priv.-Doz. Dr. med. TORSTEN ZUBERBIER
Charité-Virchow Klinikum,
Medizinische Fakultät der Humboldt-Universität zu Berlin
Dermatologische Universitätsklinik und Poliklinik
Schumannstr. 20-21, D-10117 Berlin, Germany

Priv.-Doz. Dr. med. JÜRGEN GRABBE
Medizinische Universität zu Lübeck
Klinik für Dermatologie und Venerologie
Ratzeburger Allee 160, D-23538 Lübeck, Germany

EUGENE MONROE, M.D.
Milwaukee Medical Clinic
Good Hope Road Center
3003 West Good Hope Road
Milwaukee, WI 53217, USA

ISBN-13:978-3-642-85269-5

Library of Congress Cataloging-in-Publication Data
Urtikaria. English.
Urticaria / B.M. Henz, T. Zuberbier, J. Grabbe (eds.).
p. cm.
ISBN-13:978-3-642-85269-5 e-ISBN-13:978-3-642-85267-1
DOI: 10.1007/978-3-642-85267-1

1. Urticaria. I. Henz, B.M. (Beate M.), 1941- .
II. Zuberbier, T. (Torsten), 1962- . III. Grabbe, J. (Jürgen),
1956- . IV. title.
RL249.U7813 1998
616.5'1--dc21

Softcover reprint of the hardcover 1st edition 1998

Cover design: Design & Production, Heidelberg
Typesetting: Fotosatz-Service Köhler OHG, Würzburg

SPIN: 10559213 23/3134 - 5 4 3 2 1 0 - Printed on acid-free paper

Authors

R. Brehler*

S. Chantraine-Hess

B. Cremer

I. Ehlers

J. Grabbe**

N. Haas

B.M. Henz

S. Jeep

S. Krüger-Krasagakes

A. Möller

P. Möller

E. Monroe***

W. Nürnberg

Ch. Pfrommer

T. Rosenbach

T. Zuberbier

Address of the authors: Charité-Virchow Clinics, Humboldt University, Department of Dermatology, Augustenburger Platz 1, D-13344 Berlin

* Department of Dermatology, Westfälische Wilhelms Universität, v. Esmarchstr. 56, D-48149 Münster

** Department of Dermatology, Medical University of Luebeck, Ratzeburger Allee 160, D-23538 Lübeck

*** Milwaukee Medical Clinic, Good Hope Road Center, 3003 West Good Hope Road, Milwaukee, WI 53217

Preface

Urticaria is one of the most common dermatological and allergological cutaneous reactions and, compared to other diseases, it is easily recognized by patients and physicians alike. Nevertheless, the disease is highly complex regarding its eliciting causes, its clinical manifestations and its therapy. Thus, a famous New York dermatologist once mentioned that he would rather have a lion than a patient with chronic urticaria walk into his office. This may seem surprising since, to the uninitiated, different types of urticaria look alike, and the pathomechanisms are rather well understood, with mast cells being almost invariably the main effector cells.

In 1986, a monograph of the first editor (Prof. Czarnetzki, now with the married name Henz) appeared, giving a detailed and thorough review of the then current state of knowledge regarding all aspects of the disease. Since then, two updates of this book have appeared in the German language, with coworkers of the clinic of Prof. Henz helping in the revision of the various chapters of the old monograph, and with particular emphasis on practical aspects of the disease. The present book is mainly a translation of the second German edition, with only minor updates and with more citations from the literature since the 1986 monograph is no longer available for purchase.

The editors of the previous editions of this book feel fortunate that an American collegue with particular interest in the field, Dr. Eugene Monroe from Milwaukee, USA, has joined them to help with this new English edition, particularly regarding aspects relevant to colleagues practicing medicine outside of Europe. As with the German editions, the authors have omitted complex theoretical discourses and have instead focused on practical guidelines regarding the diagnosis and therapy of urticaria, giving preference to the citation of reviews for further reading rather than to a detailed listing of older original literature.

The editors and authors have designed this book to serve as a useful guideline and reference book to dermatologists, allergologists, pediatricians and practicioners in general medicine alike, and they hope that it will provide support to the reader so that he can manage his urticaria patients more effectively.

Berlin, Lübeck and Milwaukee,

PROF. DR. MED. B. M. HENZ, M. D.
PD DR. MED. T. ZUBERBIER
PD DR. MED. J. GRABBE
E. MONROE, M. D.

Contents

1 The Spectrum of Urticaria

B.M. Henz

1.1 Historical Aspects

Urticaria was recognized as a distinct disease entity already by Hippocrates. The diverse names given to the disease by subsequent schools reflect its most important clinical aspects, namely the burning (urere), stinging and swelling (essera) on contact with nettles (urtica urens) as well as the the white discoloration (m. porcellaneus) of the wheal (Table 1.1). In the 16th century, a possible causal relationship was reported for the first time between the disease and the uptake of food proteins. The modern understanding of the disease was markedly enhanced with the discovery of the mast cell by Paul Ehrlich (1879), of histamine by Dale and Wardlaw (1910) and of IgE by Ishizaka (1966) (Czarnetzki 1989a).

Special forms of urticaria like angioedema, solar and cold urticaria as well as factitious urticaria and urticaria pigmentosa were recognized already before the beginning of the 20th century. Further subtypes like cholinergic, aquagenic and delayed pressure urticaria, intolerance reactions and urticarial

Table 1.1. Different names of urticaria in the course of history

Names	Source
Uredo	Plinius, 1st cent.
Essera (Arabic: elevation)	Hali Ben Abbas, 10th cent.
Nesselsucht (German: nettle-rash)	Valentini, 1690
Nettle rash	Hartford, 1740
Urticatio (urere, Latin: to burn)	Zedler, 1740
Randados (Spanish: nettles)	Cleghorn, 1751
Morbus porcinus (pig's disease)	Astruc, 1759
Morbus porcellaneus (porcelain disease)	Astruc, 1759
Scarlatina urticaria	Sauvages, 1763
Urticaria	Frank, 1792
Knidosis (knide: Greek: nettle)	Alibert, 1833

vasculitis were however only recognized as separate disease entities during the past decades (Czarnetzki 1989a).

1.2 Definition and Classification

Urticaria is defined by the wheal (Fig. 1.1) which is characterized by three typical aspects:

- a central whealing with surrounding reflex erythema,
- associated itching,
- its fleeting nature, with the skin returning to its normal appearance, usually within a few minutes and rarely after some hours.

Histologically, the classical fleeting wheal exhibits an edema of the epidermis and the upper and mid-dermis, with dilatation of the postcapillary venules and lymphatic vessels of the upper dermis.

Frequently, whealing is associated with more extensive swellings of the lower dermis and the subcutis. These deep swellings are called angioedema. They arise particularly frequently in skin regions where the dermis is thin and where the subcutaneous connective tissue is loosely arranged, such as in the face. Angioedema can also occur in the mucous membranes fo the upper respiratory, gastrointestinal and genitourinary tract whereas urticae are confined to the skin.

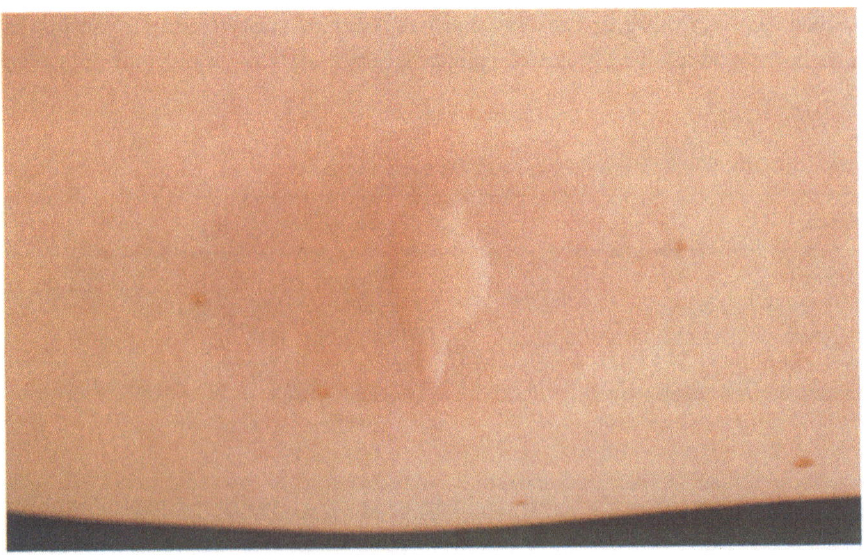

Fig. 1.1. Typical wheal with reflex erythema after injection of a histamine liberator

Table 1.2. Classification of urticaria on the basis of its duration, frequency and causes

	Duration	Frequency
a) Acute urticaria	<6 Weeks	
1. Acute continuous urticaria		Daily
2. Acute intermittent urticaria		symptomfree intervals of at least 6 wks to many months
b) Chronic urticaria	>6 Weeks	
1. Chronic continuous urticaria		Daily
2. Chronic recurrent urticaria		symptomfree intervals rangings from days to many weeks
c) Special types of urticaria		
1. Cholinergic urticaria		
2. Physical urticaria		
3. Contact urticaria		
4. Urticarial vasculitis		
5. Urticaria pigmentosa (mastocytosis)		

The spectrum of clinical manifestations of urticaria is very wide. This is due to the great diversity of eliciting causes as well as the differing reactivity of individual patients. The numerous classifications of urticaria are meant to help with the identification of the type of clinical manifestation of the individual patient, to improve understanding of the causes and the eliciting factors of the disease, and on this basis to treat the patients in a more direct and effective way.

Table 1.2 shows the classification of urticaria on the basis of its most obvious clinical aspects. The disease duration allows for its major classification into two groups, namely acute and chronic urticaria. Since acute urticaria initiated by the exposure to a stimulus at one time point resolves almost invariably after 6 weeks, this duration from the beginning of the disease is generally used as a dividing line between the two typesof urticaria. Some authors prefer to use however 4 or even 8 weeks as the line of distinction (Czarnetzki 1986; Soter 1991).

Acute urticaria is further divided into acute intermittent and acute continuous urticaria on the basis of the activity of the disease (Table 1.2). In acute intermittent urticaria, relapses occur only after 6 weeks or many months, and the eliciting agent is most likely always the same. Less than 1 % of patients with acute urticaria develop chronic urticaria (Zuberbier et al. 1995).

Chronic urticaria (Table 1.2) is also divided into a continuous type, with daily occurrence of the wheals, and a recurrent type, with whealing at intervals of several or many days. These distinctions are important in the search for the eliciting agent of the disease.

Special types of urticaria are further subdivided into several subgroups on the basis of their pathogenesis, eliciting agents and clinical aspects (Table 1.2), and they are discussed in more detail in separate chapters of this book. These types of urticaria have a chronic course and are therefore often classified as chronic urticaria. The common usage of chronic urticaria refers however generally only to the endogenous urticaria, that is the fleeting whealing reactions which are elicited systemically. Urticarial vasculitis should be differentiated from this type of chronic urticaria because the individual wheals can persist for many hours or days, due to the underlying vasculitis (see Chapter 8).

Cholinergic urticaria is often classified with physical urticaria. Since the increase in body core temperature e.g. also due to emotional stimuli and not externally applied heat is the essential eliciting factor, this entity is dealt with separately (Chapter 6).

Urticaria pigmentosa is due to an increase of mast cells in the skin and/or internal organs (mastocytosis) and can only be classified as urticaria since dermographic stimuli and histamine liberators induce whealing reactions (see Chapter 9). Contact urticaria is another special type of urticaria (Chapter 7) which is related to contact eczema because of its percutaneous elicitation and its clinical presentation. The local wheals are elicited by diverse mechanisms, and since physical stimuli also elicit whealing locally via the skin, physical urticarias (Chapter 5) should basically also be classified as contact urticaria, although this is not done in clinical practice.

Angioedemas are not mentioned in Table 1.2. They arise either together with acute or chronic urticaria, or due to defects in the inhibition of the early aspects of the complement cascade, either on the basis of diverse diseases or a genetic defect.

1.3 Pathogenesis

Because of the potential therapeutic implications, it is useful to also classify urticaria on the basis of the underlying pathomechanisms (Czarnetzki 1989b).

Classification of urticaria on the basis of its pathomechanisms
(for details see text)

A. Allergic or immunologically mediated, immunoglobulin-dependent urticaria
   1. Antigen- and antibody-induced urticaria (mostly via IgE and the FcεRI) (e.g. reactions to drugs, food, pollen; parasitosis)
   2. Factitious urticaria
   3. Cold urticaria
   4. Solar urticaria
   5. Cholinergic urticaria

B. Non-immunologic urticaria
   1. Induction by histamine liberators (s. Table 1.4)
   2. Intolerance reactions

C. Complement-mediated urticaria
   1. Hereditary angioedema
   2. Acquired angioedema
   3. Urticarial vasculitis
   4. Heat urticaria (up to 50%)
   5. Serum sickness
   6. Reactions to blood and blood products
   7. "Exercise-induced anaphylaxis" (partly)

D. Mastocytosis (urticaria pigmentosa)

E. Idiopathic urticaria

The majority of urticarial reactions are induced by stimulation of mast cells, followed by mediator release (Fig. 1.2) (Grabbe et al, 1994; Bressler 1995). Histamine is apparently the most important mediator, since most wheals after local histamine injections do not differ clinically from urticarial wheals and can also be suppressed by antihistamines. Most systemic symptoms of urticaria can also be explained by the effects of histamine. The reflex erythema of wheals is due to antidromic stimulation of free nerve endings by histamine, with subsequent release of substance P and resulting vasodilatation.

Longer lasting wheals are probably caused by chemotactic mediators from mast cells which then induce the regularly observed inflammatory infiltrate (Table 1.3). Already within a few minutes, adhesion molecules are expressed in urticarial tissue. Chemotactic lipids like leukotrienes and PAF are probably

Table 1.3. Inflammatory infiltrates or increase of cutaneous tissue resident cells in different types of urticaria

Neutrophils	Urticarial vasculitis Acute and chronic urticaria Delayed pressure urticaria
Eosinophils	Allergic urticaria Acute and chronic urticaria Delayed pressure urticaria Cholinergic urticaria
T-lymphocytes (helper type)	Persisting wheals
Mast cells	Urticaria pigmentosa All types of urticaria

responsible for the rapid immigration of neutrophils and eosinophils, while the neutrophilic, monocytic and lymphocytic (T-helper) cells of longer lasting wheals are most likely due to interleukin-8 and other chemokines, and the eosinophilic infiltrates to interleukin-5, RANTES and GM-CSF (Fig. 1.2). Mast cell products also activate complement and can thus potentially induce tissue edema, further leukocytic infiltration and additional stimulation of mast cells via the action of anaphylatoxins (e.g. C3a, C5a). C2-kinins are thought to be involved in the extensive deep tissue swellings with associated pain in hereditary angioedema (Czarnetzki 1987; Grabbe et al. 1994).

Modulation of mast cell releasability by these factors is of clinical relevance (Fig. 1.2). It is furthermore known that the surrounding tissue varies in its reactivity, depending on modulating inflammatory mediators and hormones. This might e.g. explain the worsening of chronic recurrent urticaria after viral infections or stress.

Although little is known about the role of mast cell mediators and their modulation in urticarial reactions, the mechanisms involved in the induction of urticaria have been studied extensively over several decades (Fig. 1.2). Already since the classical experiments of Prausnitz and Küstner, it is known that during passive transfer, substances contained within the serum of

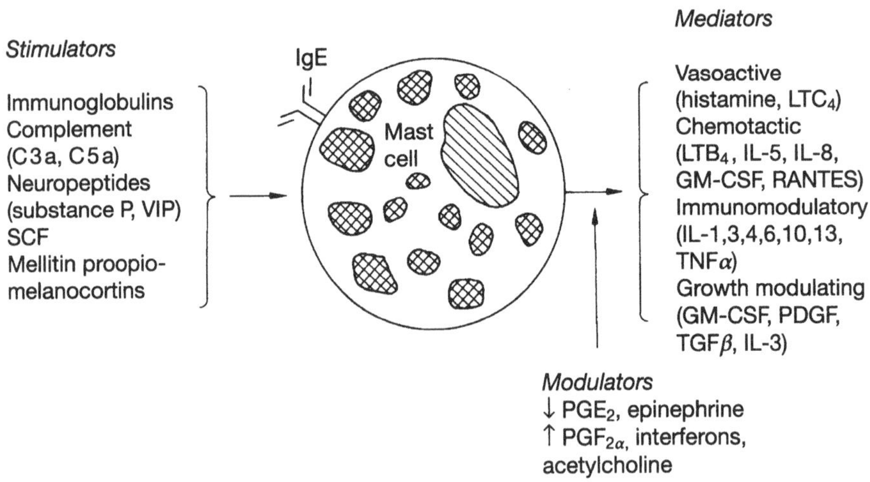

Fig. 1.2. Schematic presentation of pathomechanisms of urticaria. Mast cells are the central effector cells. They can be stimulated by diverse agents and subsequently release their mediators, particularly histamine. The intensity of this release can be stimulated (↑) or inhibited (↓) by certain modulatory substances. The listing of stimulators and mediators is only exemplary, with no claim for completeness. LT = leukotriene; IL = interleukin; TNF = tumor necrosis factor; GM-CSF = granulocyte macrophage colony stimulating factor; RANTES = *r*egulated upon *a*ctivation, *n*ormal *T* cell *e*xpressed and *s*ecreted; PDGF = platelet derived growth factor; TGF = transforming growth factor

patients bind to the skin (i.e. the mast cells) of healthy individuals, allowing for the reproduction of whealing reactions after exposure of the site to allergens or mechanical stimuli. It is now well established that this transferable serum factor is primarily antigen-specific IgE. Positive passive transfer due to IgE was also demonstrated in up to 69% of patients with cholinergic urticaria, in about one third of patients with cold urticaria, and in solar urticaria patients with reactivity in the UVB and the 400–500 nm wavelength spectrum (see also classification of urticaria, p. 13). In cold and cholinergic urticaria, other classes of immunoglobulins have been shown to mediate passive transfer as well (Czarnetzki 1989b). Recently, anti-IgE- and anti-IgE-receptor-antibodies with histamine releasing properties have been identified in a subgroup of patients with chronic urticaria (Hide et al. 1993). Numerous substances which can induce urticarial and even anaphylactic reactions independent of immunological mechanisms have also been implicated in the pathogenesis of urticaria (Table 1.4). It remains uncertain why only some persons react to these so-called histamine liberators. In patients with mastocytosis, the massive increase of mast cell numbers seems to explain however the often life threatening reactions to histamine liberators in insect venoms (mellitin, mast cell degranulating peptide) and certain drugs.

The pathomechanisms underlying increased numbers of mast cells in the skin and other organs in mastocytosis as well as in chronic urticaria are currently unclear. The increased mediator release of these cells in response to mechanical stimuli and mast cell liberators is also not well understood. Recent experimental results suggest however that growth factors from fibroblasts,

Table 1.4. Common inducers of a direct, non-immunological histamine release from mast cells

Drugs	Basic peptides	Diverse agents
Morphine	Bradykinin	Endotoxin
Codeine	Polistes	Neurotensin
Curare	Mellitin	Substance 48/80
Polymyxin B	Substance P	Acetylcholine
Dextran		Protein A
Mannitol		Formylpeptides
Chlorpromazin		Cytokines
Protamin		Concanavalin A
Enzymes	**Hormones**	**Cytotoxic stimuli**
Phospholipase A_2	ACTH	Complement
Chymotrypsin	Parathormon	Polycations
Peroxidase + H_2O_2	Somatostatin	Lysolecithin
Xanthin oxidase		Phospholipids
		Detergents

endothelial cells and keratinocytes (SCF, NGF) are potent inducers of mast cell growth, differentiation and activation (Czarnetzki et al, 1995). Increased SCF activity or an activating mutation in its receptor, the protooncogene c-kit, are probably involved in some adult patients with this disease (see Chapter 9).

Pseudoallergic intolerance reactions to aspirin, other non-steroidal antiphlogistics as well as food additives cause urticaria by non-immunological, complement-independent pathways which have so far not been clarified. In up to 50% of patients with different types of urticaria, aspirin provokes or worsens urticarial reactions (Czarnetzki 1986).

Certain complement fragments, particularly the anaphylatoxins C3a, C4a and C5a, are well known, potent mast cell liberators (Fig. 1.2). The types of urticaria induced via these molecules (see classification, Section 1.3) fail to respond to conventional antihistamines and are difficult to treat.

The last category of urticaria, the so-called idiopathic urticaria, is defined as urticaria of unknown cause. Depending on the diagnostic acumen of the physician, it is diagnosed in from 5 to 70% of patients with chronic urticaria. With the exception of infants where urticaria is mostly due to cow's milk allergy, the majority of patients with acute urticaria must also be classified with idiopathic urticaria. This represents however no major problem for the individual patient due to the transient nature of his disease.

Although urticaria can be viewed as one of the best understood diseases, there are still many open questions regarding its pathogenesis. Thus, it is not known why patients develop an immunological sensitization or an intolerance to chemical agents or physical stimuli at all. Even such simple clinical observations as the movement of wheals from one location on the skin to the other and the variably associated reaction of internal organs like the bronchial or the gastrointestinal tract are not understood. Finally, very little is known about the mechanisms which induce regression of wheals and urticarial reactions. Mast cells which are central to the pathogenesis of urticaria, should provide a fascinating model to further study the clinical and the basic aspects of this disease (Czarnetzki 1989b).

1.4 Epidemiology

Data regarding the incidence of urticaria vary widely, depending on age group, region and associated diseases (Table 1.5). The incidence in Sweden is 1.85%, with a prevalence of 0.11% for men and 0.14% for women. According to a study from Virginia, 23.6% of the general population suffer from urticaria sometime in their life. In childhood and particularly in allergic children, the prevalence is higher than in adults and it is low in old age (Czarnetzki, 1989b). Urticaria patients are seen at about equal frequency by general practicioners,

Table 1.5. Prevalence (%) of urticaria in different population groups on the basis of several studies

General population	0.05 - 0.5
Children and adolescents	2.1 - 6.7
Dermatological patients	0.8 - 4.4
Allergic patients	3.0 - 34.5
Allergic children	4.5 - 16.3
Newborns in India	23.6

family physicians and dermatological clinics (1.4–3% of all patients) (Paul and Greilich 1988). An increased incidence of urticaria has not been recorded during the past years (Haas et al. 1995).

Familial atopy is observed in only few special types of chronic urticaria. According to one study, patients with urticaria were found to have a higher risk to develop leukemia, lymphomas and myelomas (McWorter 1988, see also Section 2.5), whereas in two other studies no or even a reverse relationship was found (Vena et al. 1985; Lindelof et al. 1990).

1.5 Clinical Aspects

1.5.1 Cutaneous Manifestations

Individual wheals begin as a faint erythema which rapidly transforms into a mildly raised swelling (Fig. 1.3). Within a brief period of time, the erythema is intensified by the development of a reflex erythema at the edge of the lesion, while the raised central part develops a yellowish to white discoloration which is more apparent when the skin is spread apart. Lateral pressure on the wheal induces an orange peal-like appearance of the skin surface (see cover picture).

Wheals vary in size from tiny, pin-sized lesions which occur typically in cholinergic urticaria, to large areas of (angio)edema. In ordinary urticaria, small wheals of varying size spread and assume circular, circinate or highly irregular configurations (Figs. 1.3, 1.4, 1.5).

Very intense edema can result in blister formation on top of the wheals, particularly in children under two years of age. Wheals can also be transformed into persisting papules as is typically seen after insect bites. After resolution of the edema, a residual purpura is seen on rare occasions, particularly after the intensive inflammatory action of urticarial vasculitis (see Chapter 8).

The development of whealing is always associated with an intense pruritus which in contrast to the itch in eczema induces the patient to rub rather than excoriate the skin with his nails. The quality and intensity of itching varies

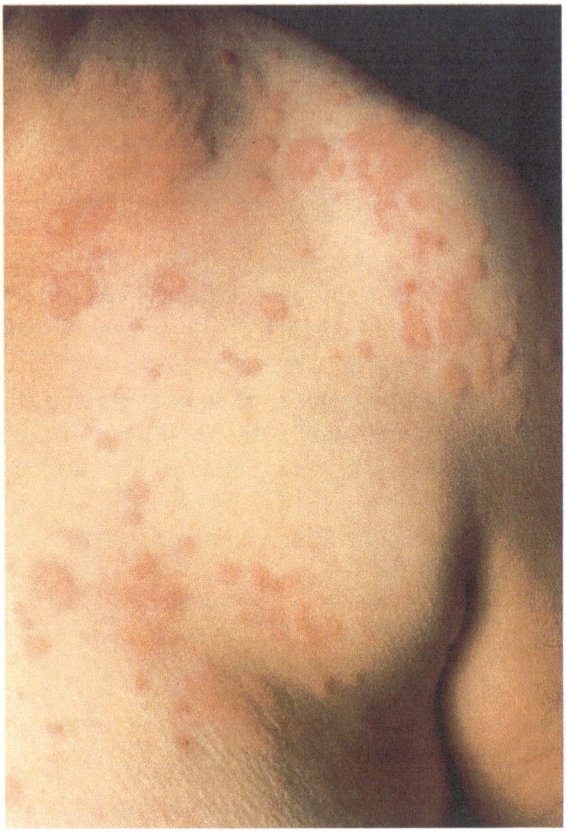

Fig. 1.3. Small wheals in a patient with a 10 year history of daily occurring, idiopathic urticaria

from patient to patient. Some patients complain about a stinging sensation, others about burning, prickling or tickling, and some fail to experience any symptoms on exposure to typically itch-inducing stimuli at all. Generally, itching of the scalp, the palms and the soles as well as over bony prominences is particularly intense. Deep swellings tend to cause pain. Most patients experience more itching in the evening and at night, particularly in a warm environment. Possible explanations are an increased mental awareness due to the lack of stimuli normally present during the day, a decreased control of the CNS due to tiredness, a drop of endogenous steroid hormone levels, an increased warmth of the skin, and an increased responsiveness of mast cells and their target tissue to eliciting stimuli. An improved vascular supply to the tissue may also allow for a more efficient transport of eliciting stimuli to the tissue in the latter case.

Individual wheals develop within seconds to minutes and vanish usually within 30 minutes to 3 hours, with the concomitant development of new lesions in adjacent or distant skin regions. The local progression of wheals can

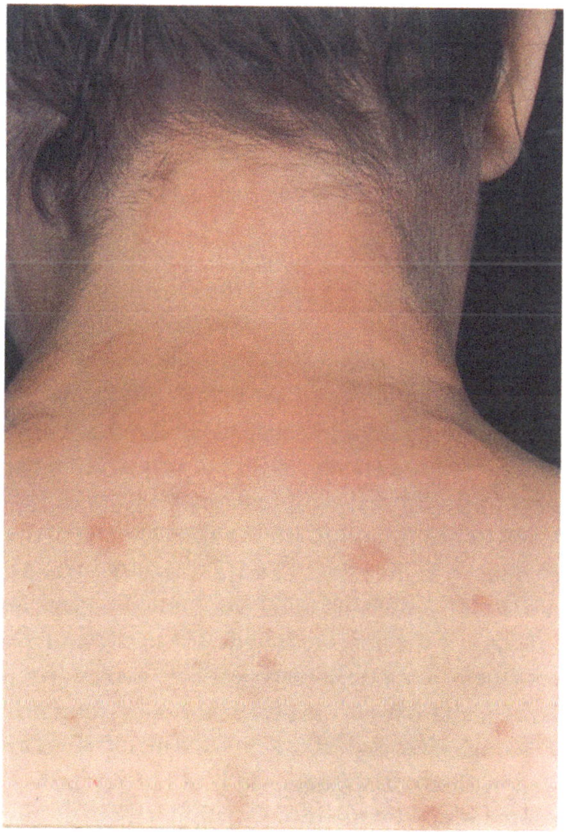

Fig. 1.4. Annular and maculopapular wheals with erythema in a patient with acute urticaria after exposure to penicillin

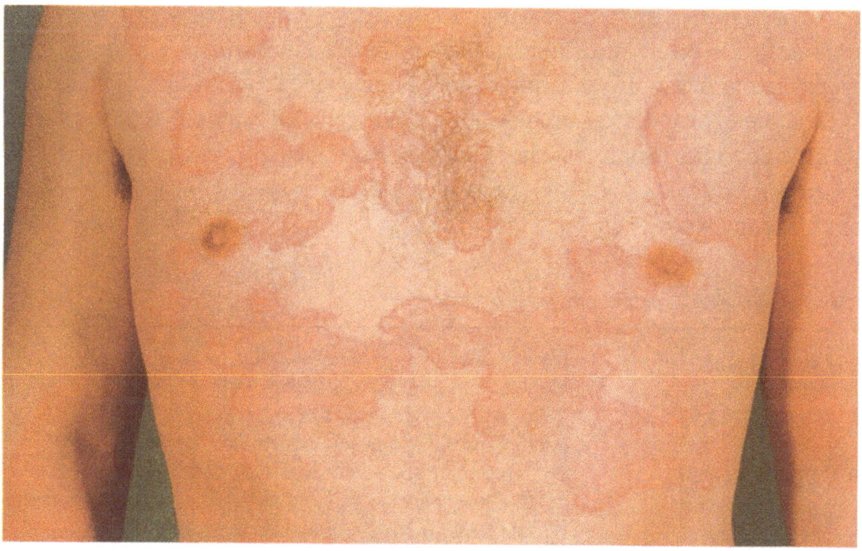

Fig. 1.5. Circinate wheals in a patient with chronic urticaria due to food intolerance

be well verified by marking the edge of the wheals with a skin marker. Most patients develop their wheals preferentially towards the end of the night, with their resolution in the course of the morning (Czarnetzki 1986; Soter 1991).

1.5.2 **Extracutaneous Symptoms** (Table 1.6)

Systemic or extracutaneous symptoms occur infrequently in acute and chronic urticaria. In view of the mostly oral or intravenous application of the eliciting stimuli, it is surprising that reactions mostly become manifest only in the skin. Other organs can be involved, via the systemic effects of mediators released by cutaneous mast cells or due to the response of mast cells in extracutaneous organs and basophils in the curculation.

In very few patients, attacks of urticaria are preceded within a few hours or days by prodromal symptoms such as loss of appetite, malaise, headache and fever. Concomitantly with the skin, allergic urticaria becomes manifest most frequently in the upper airways and the gastrointestinal tract, in the latter case particularly after the uptake of food allergens. Associated symptoms include swelling of the lips, the tongue, the palate and the throat, with dysphagia and shortness of breath. Hoarseness is an early warning sign for involvement of the larynx, and patients experiencing these symptoms are particularly anxious. Although swellings of the mucous membranes are frequently life threatening in hereditary angioedema and cold urticaria, this holds only rarely for angioedema which occurs in association with urticaria.

In asthmatics, bronchospasms and rales are often observed during a bout of urticaria. Severe asthmatic attacks can be associated with urticaria, but these symptoms are rarely recorded because of the far more worrisome respiratory symptoms, and they are accordingly rarely mentioned in the medical literature.

In acute urticaria after uptake of food allergens, patients often present with crampy abdominal pain, nausea, vomiting and diarrhea. In chronic urticaria an increase of gastric acidity can induce a gastritis, peptic ulcers or bleeding of the stomach wall.

Table 1.6. Possible systemic reactions in urticaria

1. Prodromal symptoms:	Malaise, lack of appetite, headache, fever
2. Airways:	Shortness of breath, hoarseness, asthma
3. Gastrointestinal tract:	Dysphagia, nausea, vomiting, gastritis, peptic ulcers, abdominal cramps, diarrhea
4. Nervous system:	Itching, anxiety, headache, epilepsy, hemiparesis, cerebral edema, confusion, coma (loss of hearing, ophthalmoplegia)
5. Vascular system:	Hypotension, ECG-changes, angina pectoris
6. Other:	Arthritis, fever, renal involvement, hepatitis, pancreatitis

Other possibly involved organs include the kidneys, liver and pancreas. Very rarely, patients experience cerebral edema, with headaches, epilepsy, hemiparesis, confusion and coma. Very rarely, cardiac involvement with changes of the ECG or angina due to transient ischemia are observed.

Arthritis and arthralgias are only rarely seen in association with urticaria, particularly in association with serum sickness, urticarial vasculitis, delayed pressure urticaria or systemic cold urticaria. If at all, fever is seen primarily in the latter types of urticaria and in addition with solar urticaria, angioedema associated with hypereosinophilia, malignant mastocytosis and Schnitzler's syndrome. Increased temperature can also be observed in acute and chronic urticaria in association with underlying diseases like viral infections, systemic parasitosis or malignant diseases.

Laboratory changes are rarely seen in acute and chronic urticaria and are not diagnostic or helpful, unless they are due to an underlying disease. Only rarely, a search for specific IgE is worthwhile in patients with allergic reactions to food. Whenever possible, a skin prick test should be performed instead since it is more reliable and clinically relevant (see Section 10.2.2). In some patients with acute urticaria, delayed pressure or urticarial vasculitis, neutrophilia has been observed, together with an increased ESR and rarely fever. Unexplained increases of serum IgM, serum albumin or total serum protein have been observed in up to 50% of patients with chronic urticaria. Total serum IgE is increased in only up to 13% of patients. Decreased complement levels can be observed particularly in urticarial vasculitis.

1.5.3 Anaphylaxis

In highly sensitized patients with type I allergies, or even in weakly sensitized patients after parenteral application of the allergen, anaphylactic shock can develop with or without associated urticaria. The reaction develops rapidly and reaches its maximum within 5–30 minutes. Initially, the patients may experience itching on palms and soles, in the genital region or the external auditory meatus. Others note a prickling sensation on tongue and palate, nausea, substernal pressure or dyspnea. Further symptoms associated with hypotension include bronchospasms, laryngeal edema, urticaria, angioedema, diffuse erythema, cardiac arrhythmias and increased intestinal mobility. In contrast to animals where the primary shock organ is very consistent, namely the lung in guinea pigs and the gastrointestinal tract in dogs, the anaphylactic symptomatology of humans is unpredictable and highly variable.

In patients with bee and wasp venom allergies, it has been reported that associated urticaria is often a sign for less life threatening anaphylactic reactions. This is however not invariably so. In patients with very prominent anaphylactic reactions, urticarial symptoms sometimes arise only many hours later, after resolution of the acute symptoms.

1.5.4 Serum Sickness

This condition develops whenever antigens persist for protracted periods in the serum and allow for the formation of immune complexes. The cutaneous lesions are maculopapular rather than urticarial. They are more frequent and marked at the sites of injections, but may also be generalized. In addition, one can observe fever, lymphadenopathy, arthritis, nephritis, angioedema, neuritis and severe gastrointestinal symptoms, as well as a leukocytosis, an increased ESR and a mild eosinophilia.

Serum sickness has become less frequent with the decrease of therapeutic use of foreign serum and immunoglobulin injections. Currently, antibiotics, sulfonamides, antiepileptic drugs or radio contrast media are more likely causes. After the first exposure, an interval of at least 5–7 days is necessary for the development of sufficient quantities of antibodies to allow for immune complex formation. After repeated injections, symptoms develop more rapidly, and fulminant reactions are associated with diarrhea, asthma, epileptic attacks, shock, coma and finally death. Generally, symptoms abate in dependence of the elimination half life of the eliciting antigen within a few days or weeks.

1.6 Clinical Aspects of Intolerance Reactions

Hirschberg (1902) was the first to describe an intolerance reaction in a patient whom he had treated with aspirin for arthralgias. His description of the clinical symptoms are classical for aspirin intolerance.

> "... at 7 p.m., I gave the patient 1 g of aspirin which I had learned to appreciate as an excellent treatment for pain, rheumatic and nervous conditions.
>
> Towards 10 p.m., the patient complained of marked swellings of his face, particularly his eyes and his lower lips, and his nose appeared occluded. He complained of mucosa exudates in his pharynx which he could only remove with continuous clearence of the throat. His scalp was swollen and itchy, he experienced difficulties in speaking, and he was generally apathic.
>
> On my arrival, he presented with the following symptoms: Both eyelids were grossly swollen so that his eyes could be only opened to a narrow slit. His lower lip was swollen, the mucous membranes were edematous and hypererythematous. The swollen lids and the lower lip were hard and infiltrated on palpation.
>
> ... I attribute his symptoms to an unwanted effect of aspirin since no other cause could be found and since other possible causes (ingestion of crabs or strawberries) had not been present. One must therefore assume in this case an unexplainable idiosyncratic reaction of the patient to aspirin."

Pseudoallergic reactions to acetylsalicylic acid in patients with preexisting chronic urticaria or asthma generally induce an acute worsening of the basic disease (Ros et al. 1976).

Patients without underlying disease can react with urticaria, angioedema or bronchospasms. Typical symptoms of the latter patients are also erythema of the face (Fig. 1.6).

Dizziness, headache, tiredness, tachycardia, palpitations, diffuse sweating and gastrointestinal disturbances are frequently associated symptoms. Fulminant reactions with fever, cramps or anaphylactic shock can occur, but fortunately rarely.

In about half of the patients, this symptomatology occurs within 6 hours after exposure to the eliciting agent (Juhlin 1981). The latency period can however reach from a few minutes up to 24 hours. Cutaneous symptoms have a longer latency than systemic reactions.

Most of the symptoms disappear after one or two days. Particularly after ingestion of acetylsalicylic acid, urticarial reactions can, however, persist for 1-2 weeks.

After the symptoms have disappeared, there is an individually variable refractory period for up to 72 hours. During this time, the patients tolerate all types of substances which they normally react to. This explains why substances which are taken regularly in small quantities on a daily basis general-

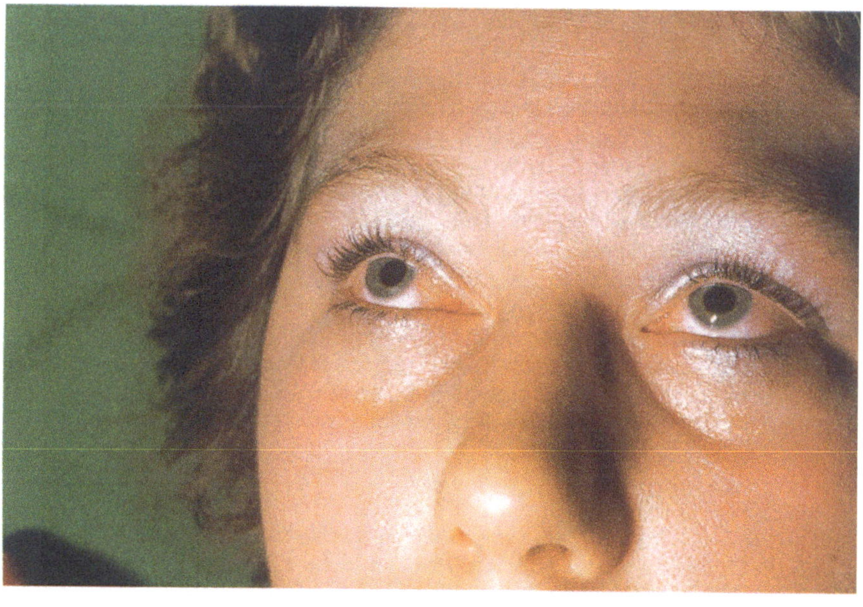

Fig. 1.6. Intolerance reaction after ingestion of aspirin. Note the facial erythema, the redness of the conjunctiva and the periorbital edema

ly cause only mild reactions, with acute and particularly vehement reactions after they have been avoided for a while. If the eliciting agents are avoided for 1/2 to 1 year, the reactivity may however disappear entirely, without future recurrences.

Pseudoallergic reactions thus have a clear tendency to spontaneous remission. About 30% of patients with proven aspirin intolerance on oral provocation fail to react after reexposure one year later (Ros et al. 1976; Paul et al. 1994).

According to Wüthrich (1983), one should differentiate between intolerance reactions and intolerance provocation. The latter would involve the aggravation of an existing disease on exposure to the pseudoallergen, while intolerance reactions would induce the symptomatology in otherwise normal individuals. These two types of conditions can also be distinguished in patients with chronic urticaria.

Literature

Bressler RB (1995) Pathophysiology of chronic urticaria. Im All Clinics N Am 15:659-677

Czarnetzki BM (1986) Urticaria, Springer, Berlin Heidelberg New York Tokyo

Czarnetzki BM (1987) Mechanisms and mediators in urticaria. Sem Dermatol 6:272-285

Czarnetzki BM (1989a) History of urticaria. Int J Dermatol 28:52-57

Czarnetzki BM (1989b) Urticaria. In: Norris D (ed) Immune mechanisms in cutaneous disease. Dekker, New York, pp 653-670

Czarnetzki BM, Grabbe J, Kolde G, Krüger-Krasagakes S, Zuberbier T (1995) Mast cells in the cytokine network - the what, where from and what for. Exp Dermatol 4:221-226

Grabbe J, Haas N, Czarnetzki BM (1994) Die Mastzelle. Hautarzt 45:55-64

Haas N, Klapproth I, Czarnetzki BM (1995) Vergleichende Studie zur Häufigkeit, Diagnostik und Therapie der Urtikaria in einer Hautpoliklinik. Allergologie 18:110-113

Hide M, Francis DM, Grattan CEH, Hakimi J, Kochan JP, Greaves MW (1993) Autoantibodies against the high-affinity IgE receptor as a cause of histamine release in chronic urticaria. N Engl J Med 328:1599-1604

Hirschberg L (1902) Mittheilung über einen Fall von Nebenwirkung des Aspirins. Dtsch Med Wochenschr 23:416

Juhlin L (1981) Recurrent urticaria: clinical investigation of 330 patients. Br J Dermatol 104: 369-381

Lindelof B, Sigurgeirsson B, Wahlgren CF, Eklund G (1990) Chronic urticaria and cancer: An epidemiological study of 1155 patients. Br J Dermatol 128:453-456

McWorter WP (1989) Allergy and risk of cancer. A prospective study using NHANESI follow-up data. Cancer 64:451-455

Paul E, Greilich K-D (1991) Zur Epidemiologie der Urtikaria-Erkrankungen. Hautarzt 42: 366-375

Paul E, Geipel M, Möller R (1994) Katamnestische Untersuchungen an Patienten mit chronischer Urtikaria und ASS-Intoleranz. Hautarzt 45:12-14

Ros AM, Juhlin L, Michaelsson G (1976) A follow-up study of patients with recurrent urticaria and hypersensitivity to aspirin, benzoates and azo dyes. Br J Dermatol 95: 19-24

Soter NA (1991) Acute and chronic urticaria and angioedema. J Am Acad Dermatol 25: 146-154
Vena JE, Bona JR, Byers TE, Middleton E Jr, Swanson MK, Graham S (1985) Allergy-related diseases and cancer: An inverse association. Am J Epidemiol 122:66-74
Wüthrich B (1983) Allergische und pseudoallergische Reaktionen der Haut durch Arzneimittel und Lebensmitteladditiva. Schweiz Rundsch Med (PRAXIS) 72:691-699
Zuberbier T, Iffländer J, Semmler C, Czarnetzki BM (1996) Acute urticaria - clinical aspects and therapeutic responsiveness. Acta Derm Venereol (Stockh) 76:295-297

2 Causes of Urticaria

B. M. Henz and T. Zuberbier

2.1 General Aspects

Strictly speaking, the reasons why otherwise healthy persons develop an allergy or intolerance to substances in their external or internal environment with resulting urticarial reactions, are largely unclear. Genetic factors play hardly any role since only rare types of urticaria are familial. Associated viral infections, as they are often observed in acute urticaria (Zuberbier et al. 1996), might represent a triggering factor, but the possible mechanisms are poorly understood (see also Section 2.2.1).

This chapter will deal therefore primarily with the eliciting factors of whealing reactions (Table 2.1). These encompass a broad range of agents which induce mast cell release via a similarly wide spectrum of mechanisms. The eliciting stimuli reach dermal mast cells either in form of exogenous allergens, pseudoallergens or infectious agents and their products or they are produced by the body itself e.g. in the course of internal diseases.

Table 2.1. Major categories of stimuli or causes of urticarial reactions

- Food proteins, preservatives, colorants
- Drugs
- Inhalant allergens
- Contactants (see Chapter 7)
- Infections and infestations
- Internal diseases
- Malignencies
- Hormones
- Physical and mental stress (see Chapter 6)
- Physical agents (see Chapter 5)

2.2 Allergic Urticaria

2.2.1 Pathomechanisms

Except for infants and young children, specific pathological hyperreactions of the immune system, i.e. type I allergic reactions, can be identified in only a small number of patients with acute and chronic urticaria. Besides type I allergic reactions, immune complexes containing IgE and other types of immunoglobulins can be involved, with associated complement activation (Czarnetzki 1986, 1989). Recently, the induction of urticaria via autoantibodies of different types has been discussed, with those against the α-chain of the high affinity IgE receptor being particularly interesting (Hide et al. 1993). These autoantibodies are however probably a secondary phenomenon since they are also present in 40% of patients with pseudoallergy to food ingredients who respond to a diet (unpublished own observations).

Strictly speaking, urticarial vasculitis should be classified with allergic urticaria; it is however dealt with separately in this book because of its many special features (Chapter 8). The same holds for contact urticaria (Chapter 7) and several types of physical urticaria (Chapter 5) since immunological and specific allergic pathomechanisms play a role in these conditions as well.

In allergic urticaria, a sensitization of the immune system has taken place against a defined substance. This allergen is first taken up and processed by immunocompetent dendritic cells which in turn pass the processed antigen on to lymphocytes. The latter proliferate, differentiate and finally produce immunoglobulins against the antigen during the subsequent 7–10 days. Of all immunoglobulin classes, IgE is most frequently involved in urticaria. It is a cytophylic antibody which binds with high specificity to receptors on mast cells, basophil leukocytes and Langerhans cells (Sutton and Gould, 1993).

On renewed contact with the specific allergen, the cells, mainly mast cells in urticaria, secrete their mediators, and the body reacts with allergic symptoms which range from minimal reactions on skin and mucous membranes to fulminant anaphylactic shock. These same reactions can also be initiated after histamine secretion subsequent to complement activation via immune complexes, or through mast cell releasing factors which can be generated during immunological processes or via neurological activation and hormonal secretion (Grabbe et al, 1994).

It is presently not known why only certain persons develop sensitization after allergen exposure. Genetic factors and the nature of the antigen may play a role. Furthermore, IgE production is induced and enhanced through certain interleukins (IL-4, -6, -13), viral infections (e.g. RSV, EBV), drugs (e.g. retinoids) and possibly also through environmental factors like cigarette smoke and diesel exhaust (Czarnetzki, 1989). The allergic response is increased with repeated antigen contact, and it decreases or even disappears entirely with time after allergen avoidance. Prick test reactions to penicillin were detectable in only 10% of patients after 5–10 years when the allergen was carefully avoided (Finke et al. 1965). Most patients lose their urticaria within 5 years (Lin, 1992).

2.2.2 Routes of Elicitation

Urticarial reactions are not only elicited by diverse allergens, but also via divergent pathways (Table 2.2). Orally or systemically applied drugs are the most frequent causes of allergic urticarial reactions in adults. In children, urticaria is elicited in 44% by food, followed by infections. An elicitation of urticaria by inhalation is relatively rare and is observed primarily in highly sensitized atopics. Equally rarely, urticaria is observed after vaginal or rectal application of allergens or due to antigens formed within the body in the course of chronic inflammatory diseases or malignancies. In the latter situation, urticaria assumes a chronic course before its cause is recognized. Urticaria can also be elicited after direct application of allergens or unspecific stimulants to the skin. The resulting so-called contact urticaria is dealt with in separate chapters (see Chapters 5 and 7).

Table 2.2. Diverse routes of elicitation and causes of urticarial reactions

Route of elicitation	Elicitors
Oral	Drugs
	Food
Parenteral	Drugs
	Vaccines
	Insect venoms
Inhalation	Pollen
	Allergen-containing dust
	Perfumes
Vaginal/rectal	Drugs
	Seminal fluid
	Latex
Endogenous	Bacterial toxins
	Bacterial, viral and parasite proteins
	Implants
	Hormones
	Autoantibodies
	Modified body proteins
Transcutaneous (also airborne)	Drugs
	Perfumes

2.2.3 Drugs

Allergic mechanisms are involved in less than 25% of drug reactions and become clinically manifest as urticaria, angioedema and rarely as anaphylactic shock. Drug reactions present mostly as maculopapular morbilliform or urticarial rashes, although mixed types of reactions can occur as well.

Antibiotics are the most frequent cause of anaphylactic reactions (Table 2.3), with penicillin being most frequent. Up to 7% of the general population are sensitized, according to the literature, and urticaria accounts for up to 40% of penicillin reactions (Speer et al. 1978). Depending on the route of administration and the degree of sensitization, clinical reactions can develop extremely rapidly, that is within 2–20 minutes. Delayed urticarial reactions that develop only after 2–20 hours are less threatening since they are only rarely associated with laryngeal edema and shock. Late reactions of the serum sickness type present, as already described, a mixed clinical picture. In case IgE antibodies are simultaneously present, associated increased immune complex deposition in the vessel walls after vasodilatation due to histamine can worsen the clinical picture.

Anaphylactic reactions due to penicillin can be elicited by the molecule itself or by diverse components of the preparations. The major antigen is penicilloyl (95%); other so-called minor antigens, namely penicilloate, penilloate and penicillamine, can be generated as degradation products during the process of fermentation. In biosynthetic and semisynthetic penicillin preparations, higher molecular weight impurities have additionally been identified. The newer semisynthetic penicillins may cause sensitization against the β-lactame structure and thus cross-reactions with other antibiotics carrying

Table 2.3. Causes of urticaria in patients with drug reactions (frequent examples)

Penicillin and other antibiotics	Antidiabetic drugs
Sulfonamides	Thyroid drugs
Antituberculous drugs	Vaccines
Acyclovir	Antigen extracts for hyposensitization
Thiabendazol	Amiodarone
Antiphlogistic and analgetic drugs	Procainamide
Sedatives and hypnotics	Blood products and substitutes
Carbamazepin	Heparin
Ethosuximide	Monoclonal antibodies
Diuretics and laxatives	Cytokines, interferons
Contraceptives	Antihistamines
Local anesthetics	Corticosteroids
	ACE inhibitors

this structure, but also isolated allergies against the different side chains. To a lesser extent, crossreactions are observed with different cephalosporins (up to 17%), but they are frequent with carbepenems (50%) and penicillamine (40-60%) (Saxon et al. 1988). Rare urticarial reactions to ampicillin are due to a specific allergy against the molecule, while the pathogenesis of the more frequent morbilliform type of ampicillin rash is unclear.

The high incidence of penicillin allergy is thus most likely due to the antigenicity of the molecules contained in the preparation, as well as to the diversity of its allergens and the frequent use of this potent and valuable drug. Furthermore, the molecule is very stable, also against boiling and sterilisation with hot steam. For that reason, hidden traces of the substance in milk products, meat and even in non-alcoholic beverages can lead to an unrecognized sensitization and to the maintenance of chronic urticaria (Omerod et al. 1987). Patients must therefore also be observed for at least one hour even after a first penicillin treatment so that shock reactions in patients sensitized by unknown pathways can promptly be treated.

Other antibodies inducing urticaria (Table 2.3) are tetracyclines, sulfonamides, griseofulvin, streptomycin, rifampicin and chloramphenicol. Diuretics and laxatives, particularly plant extracts, are also frequent causes. Contraceptives, vaccines, blood products, heparin, enzymes, anxiolytics, hypnotics, fibrin, formaldehyde and plasma expanders are on the other hand only rarely implicated (Cardot et al. 1995; McGrath et al. 1985; Odeh and Oliven 1992; Wantke et al. 1995; Wüthrich et al. 1996). With the more frequent therapeutic use of monoclonal antibodies or cytokines like IL-2, GM-CSF and interferons, allergic reactions with urticaria to these molecules are increasingly being reported. Orthopedic or orthodontic implantations (tantalium, platinum) can rarely act as allergens either by themselves or by complexing with body proteins. Reactions can also be due to added agents like antibiotics. It is furthermore easily overseen that even antihistamines and corticosteroids can rarely cause IgE dependent allergic reactions.

Nonsteroidal antiphlogistics, local anesthetics and radiocontrast media cause urticaria by non-immunological, as yet largely unclear mechanisms (see Section 2.3). The same holds for plasma expanders, opiates, chinin and curare which act as direct histamine liberators and which are particularly dangerous in patients with mastocytosis (see Chapter 9). Only 50% of drug reactions during anesthesia are IgE-mediated (Cardol et al. 1995).

Treatment with digestive enzymes can also cause urticarial reactions, but chymotrypsin- and dehydrocholic acid-containing preparations act also as direct histamine liberators.

After blood transfusions, urticarial reactions are caused by immune complexes, e.g. through aggregated IgG, and subsequent complement activation. Anti-IgA-antibodies develop preferentially after immunoglobulin injections.

2.2.4 Inhalent Allergens

Urticarial reactions to inhaled substances are relatively rare. Instead, asthma and rhinitis are the most common manifestations at the primary organs of contact. Reactions are particularly frequent in highly sensitized patients with pollen- and drug-allergies, professionally exposed workers and smokers.

In patients with pollen allergies, urticaria is most frequent during the pollen season. The most important allergens are tree and grass pollens. Some patients also develop urticaria after nasal provocation. During a successful hyposensitization for allergic rhinitis, the associated urticaria can disappear as well.

Up to 5% of workers in flour industries develop urticaria via inhalation. Besides the allergy to meal dust, a high percentage of these patients react also to mite allergens during skin test. In industrial workers, urticaria via inhalation is also observed from beans, platinum, aliphatic polyamines, spices, penicillin, ammonia, sulfur dioxide, formaldehyde, sodium sulfide, aminothiazide and lindane.

Apart from industrial and professional exposure, reactions to inhalent allergens can rarely also occur in daily life. Thus, highly allergic patients may even react to the smell of fried fish eaten by others (Crespo et al. 1995).

Cigarettes can induce urticaria as well, with three different allergens being so far identified. In cigarette smoke and in aqueous extracts of cured tobacco leaves, an 18 kD glycoprotein has been found that causes positive skin test reactions in one-third of smokers and nonsmokers. It is unclear whether this molecule causes IgE-mediated allergies. It crossreacts with other members of the Solanaceae family, such as green and red peppers, eggplant, potato and tomato. The clinical significance of this allergen as elicitor of urticaria is as yet unclear (Becker et al. 1976). An urticaria to glycerin in tobacco smoke was however clearly documented, with a corresponding positive skin test. The patient tolerated cigarettes which contained aliphatic aldehydes or diethylene glycerin without any problems (Rappaport and Hoffman 1941).

Other allergens from the group of aliphatic aldehydes are formaldehyde and acrolein, which are frequently found in fried and cooked food, in garlic and in frequently used oily extracts. Menthol is another allergen that is added to many types of cigarettes and can cause urticaria. It is also present in aerosoles, cough lozenges, paper handkerchiefs and skin creams (McGowen 1966).

In recent years, numerous reports have been published on urticarial and anaphylactic reactions to latex-containing gloves or latex-containing dust particles in hospitals, particular in operating rooms. Latex is also of major importance in the development of contact urticaria (see Chapter 7). In some patients, reactions to ethylene dioxide which are probably not IgE-mediated have also occured during hemodialysis.

2.2.5 Food

Chronic urticaria due to intolerance reactions to food is mostly based on pseudoallergic mechanisms. In acute urticaria, IgE-mediated type I allergic reactions are rare but must be ruled out in case of ingestion of possible allergens shortly before onset of urticaria. Reactions to food are caused by allergens that are acid-resistant, 18–36 kD glycoproteins (Table 2.4) and are associated with IgE as well as IgG production to allergens, with the latter having no pathological significance (Sampson and Metcalfe 1992; Wüthrich 1988; Zuberbier and Czarnetzki 1992, 1993). Some allergens, like those in fresh apples, are destroyed by cooking. Food also contains substances which cause histamine release via non-immunological mechanisms, or they induce clinical symptoms due to vasoactive amines or other pharmacological agents (Table 2.5, see also Section 2.3). These substances can also increase the permeability of the intestines to allergens and thus potentially enhance an allergic reaction.

Children of atopic parents suffer twice as frequently from food-induced allergies (58%), compared to children with only one parent or none being genetically predisposed (29% and 13% respectively). Allergy to cow's milk and egg tends to disappear spontaneously, mostly by the third birthday, even though skin tests remain positive for some years. It is more likely to persist with fish and peanut (Boch 1987). In older children and adults, the frequency of certain food allergies depends on the eating habits. Thus, in central Europe, allergies to spices are particular frequent whereas in Japan and Scandinavia, allergies to different types of fish and in the US, peanut allergy are predominant. There are well-known crossreactivities between foods of the Umbelliferae family (beets, cellary, mugwort), and some patients also crossreact to carrots, potatoes, apples and tomatoes. Crossreactions between fresh fruits, nuts, spices and birch pollen may occur as well (Wüthrich 1988).

Table 2.4. Known allergens in important foods

Food	Allergens
Milk	Casein, α- and β-lactalbumin, albumin
Egg white	Ovalbumin, ovomucoid, ovotransferrin
Egg yolk	Lipoprotein, livetin, several unknown fractions
Cereals (wheat)	Glutelin, albumin, globulin, gliadin
Rice	Glutelin, globulin
Tomatoes	Several glycoproteins

Table 2.5. Examples of foods that cause urticarial reactions via IgE-mediated mechanisms, directly through vasoactive amines within food or via pharmacological or other mechanisms. (Individual foods can also cause urticaria via several mechanisms.)

IgE-mediated	Vasoactive amines	Other mechanisms
Fish	Cheese	Plums
Crustaceans	Beer	Beans (especially soye)
Milk	Wine	Coffein
Nuts	Sausage	Onions
Beans	Fish	Melons
Potatoes	Conserved food	Citrus fruits
Cellery	Ananas	Tomatoes
Parsley	Avocado	Strawberries
Cereals	Meat	Mushrooms
Rice	Sauerkraut	Yeasts
Bananas	Bananas	Aliphatic aldehydes
Oranges		Azo dyes
Apples		Benzoic acid derivatives
Pollen		Salicylates
Chocolate		Menthol
Vegetables		Alcohol (ethanol)
Carrageenan		Glutamate, aspartame
		Sulfites

Examples for hidden foods are pollen in honey as well as fish allergens in cod-liver oil. The latter may also be added to sauces or be contained in meat from poultry or pigs which were fed fish meal, in glues and possibly also in wine since in France, fish-albumin is used to clear the wine. Furthermore, allergens contained in soye, beans and peanuts may be added to certain types of chocolate as a milk substitute, and guar gum is used for the thickening of sauces and milk products. Rare nonimmunological eliciting agents of urticaria in food are aliphatic aldehydes in garlic and menthol in sweets and ice tea (Warin and Champion 1974.

On oral provocation tests, the skin is the most frequent reactive organ, with urticarial and morbilliform rashes (74%), followed by gastrointestinal (43%) and respiratory (28%) symptoms. Clinical reactions that occur within the first 45 minutes are usually urticarial and IgE-mediated. They can already become manifest as local itching and swelling on contact with the lips. Delayed type reactions (1–20 hours) can also be IgE-mediated, either due to the duration of time needed for the food to pass through stomach and intestines where it is converted to an allergen by the digestive process, or on the basis of well-known late phase, IgE-mediated reactions. The predominant clinical manifestations of food allergy are gastrointestinal symptoms like vomiting and diarrhea. Delayed reactions occuring after more than 20 hours elicit intestinal symptoms and/or cutaneous eczema. Fish, berries, nuts and egg white preferentially cause immediate type reactions whereas cereals, milk, egg yolk, chocolate and nuts elicit mainly late phase reactions. Some patients have noted a refractory period of several hours after their symptoms have abated.

2.3 Pseudoallergies

2.3.1 Definitions

Pseudoallergy is a nonimmunologically mediated disease which clinically mostly mimics immediate type allergic reactions. The clinical reactions are also called anaphylactoid reactions and incorrectly also intolerance reactions, since this term should strictly speaking be reserved for pharmacological intolerance. The term pseudoallergic reactions (PAR) has been coined as a collective term for all nonimmunologically mediated reactions to certain substances (Schlumberger 1983; Schlumberger 1974). PAR can imitate all four types of allergic reactions according to Coombs and Gell. Anaphylactoid reactions can also be classified as PAR corresponding clinically to type I allergy. On the basis of its nonimmunological character, the reaction can occur already on first contact with the elicitor, without a sensitization period. Most pseudoallergic reactions are however elicited by substances which have been tolerated over many years. The basic characteristics of these reactions can be summarized as follows:

Table 2.6. Characteristic of pseudoallergic reactions

- Clinical manifestations mimic type I allergies
- Non IgE-mediated
- Dose-dependent
- Symptoms possible already on first contact with the elicitor
- Reactions also to chemically non-related substances
- Skin tests are irrelevant
- In vitro tests are not available

2.3.2 Classification and Frequency

Pseudoallergic reactions are an important pathogenetic factor in acute and particularly also in chronic urticaria. The best known reaction of this type is that due to aspirin and other nonsteroidal antiphlogistics. Other eliciting

Table 2.7. Agents causing pseudoallergic reactions

- Antiphlogistics (particularly aspirin)
- Food additives
- Natural agents in food (salicylates, benzoates, etc.)
- Radiocontrast media
- Colloidal plasma expanders
- Local anesthetics
- Diverse drugs

agents, particularly of chronic urticaria, are naturally occurring food ingredients or additives.

Further well known intolerance reactions are due to radiocontrast media, colloidal plasma expanders, anesthetics and a heterogeneous group of drugs.

Pseudoallergic reactions must be distinguished from reactions due to a group of substances which cause a direct release of histamine. These so-called histamine liberators can induce clinical symptoms resembling type I allergies. The reactions occur however in each exposed person, in contrast to PAR which represent a pathological reaction of specific individuals to generally tolerated agents.

Histamine liberators have been discussed as elicitors of acute urticaria in Chapter 1 and have been listed in Table 1.4. Poisonous reactions after the uptake of histamine-contaminated food must also be differentiated from intolerance reactions. In these situations, histamine is generated as a bacterial breakdown product of histidin and is found at highest concentrations in fish of the scombroidae family (tuna, mackerel) that has not been properly processed.

Intolerance reactions can be distinguished according to their primary organ manifestation:

- One group of patients reacts primarily with bronchoconstriction, and in case of preexisting asthma, this is acutely worsened. 10% of these patients also develop urticaria and/or angioedema.
- A second group of patients reacts primarily with cutaneous symptoms, particularly urticaria and angioedema. Symptoms may be restricted to acute urticaria, possibly associated with shortness of breath. They may also present as a worsening of preexisting chronic urticaria, and they may similarly precipitate or worsen atopic eczema. Wüthrich has proposed that the worsening of a preexisting disease should be called "intolerance provocation" (Wüthrich 1983).
- Further organ manifestations involve the gastrointestinal tract and the upper respiratory tract. Associated systemic symptoms are also possible. The worst reaction is anaphylactoid shock which is just as life threatening as that due to IgE-mediated reactions.

2.3.3 Epidemiology

Unfortunately, there are hardly any reliable data available regarding the incidence or prevalence of pseudoallergic urticarial reactions since most studies are retrospective, and very often, inclusion criteria regarding the kind of urticaria are not clearly defined. This may explain the large discrepancies between different studies.

The frequency of urticarial intolerance reactions in relation to the most frequent eliciting agents summarized in Table 2.5 which gives mean values of different studies but should be regarded as only a rough estimate of true frequencies. There is an increased incidence in patients with chronic urticaria and in patients with the so-called aspirin triade (intrinsic asthma, nasal polyps, aspirin intolerance, i.e. the so-called Samter-Syndrome). Patients who present solely with chronic rhinitis have no increased risk of intolerance reactions, compared to the normal population.

Urticarial reactions to aspirin are more frequent in adults than in children, with a peak incidence in the 2nd and 4th decade. There are no data suggesting an increased incidence of atopic diseases in the patient or family history (Schlumberger 1983).

The severity of intolerance reactions varies considerably, and only a minor fraction is life threatening. In case of radiocontrast media, for example, the incidence of urticarial reactions is 2–8%, that of life threatening reactions however less than 0.1% (Liebermann 1991), but all in all, the incidence is decreasing with the use of modern, better tolerated contrast media.

Table 2.8. Incidence of pseudoallergic urticarial reactions (means of values from diverse authors)

Eliciting agent		Incidence (%)
1. Aspirin intolerance		
a) Patients with urticaria		50
b) Asthmatics		7
c) Patients with chronic rhinitis		1.5
d) Normal population	adults	3.8
	children	0.3
2. Food additives		
a) Patients with urticaria		40
b) Asthmatics		18
3. Radiocontrast media		
a) Ionic, highly hyperosmolar		8
b) Non-ionic, less hyperosmolar		2
4. Diverse eliciting agents		
Local and intravenous anesthetics		0.5
Gelatin		8

2.4 Infections and Infestations

Despite their high frequency, bacteria only rarely cause urticarial reactions, probably since they induce IgG rather than IgE synthesis. In addition, there is probably also an increased allergic tolerance in the adult population because of previous frequent and intense exposure, whereas children still exhibit relatively frequent reactions.

Only few bacteria have been implicated as possible causes of urticaria (Table 2.9). An association between urticaria and borreliosis has been reported so far only once (Olson and Esterly 1990). Three types of bacterial infections seem to be more frequently associated with urticaria: 1. Streptococcal tonsillitis in children, 2. chronic sinusitis and dental abscesses in adolescents and adults, and 3. helicobacter infections in patients with upper abdominal pain (Möller et al. 1995). In the first situation, proof for a causative role of streptococcal antigens has so far not been provided. Treatment of sinus disease and dental abscesses is however associated with resolution of urticaria in 30% of patients. In patients with helicobacter-pylori-infections, these numbers are even higher (Möller et al. 1995, Tebbe et al. 1996). In the recently described Cogan-syndrome (urticarial vasculitis, vestibuloacustic dysfunction, superficial keratitis), antibodies against Chlamydia trachomatis have been identified, but their causative role remains unclear (Ochinsky, 1991).

The most important viral infections regarding their frequency are probably upper respiratory tract infections which are found to be responsible for approximately 40% of acute urticaria cases in adults (Zuberbier et al. 1996). Among other viral infections, hepatitis-B viruses are most frequently mentioned as a cause of urticaria. Up to 30% of patients develop urticarial rashes during the prodromal phase, together with serum sickness-like symptoms. During hepatitis-B-viremia, urticaria can be associated with necrotizing vasculitis, fever, arthralgias, mononeuritis multiplex, abdominal cramps and renal involvement. 15.3% of patients with urticaria have been found to have serum antibodies against the hepatitis-B-surface antigen, and the antigen itself was found in 2.4% (Vaida et al. 1983) The histological hallmark is a necrotizing venulitis. More recently, hepatitis C virus has also been implicated as a cause of urticaria (Kanazawa et al. 1996).

Infectious mononucleosis is a further frequent cause of urticaria (5% incidence), and urticaria can already be manifest during the incubation period, up to two weeks before the appearance of clinical manifestations. Other viruses, including the HIV virus (Friedman et al. 1995), have been described as possibly primary causative agents (Table 2.8), although they most frequently exacerbate an already preexisting urticaria, which also holds for upper respiratory tract infection patients with chronic urticaria.

Fungal infections as a cause of urticaria are considered mainly to be due to candida, with the exception of three well documented cases in the literature where a tinea pedis infection due to Trichophyton rubrum was the cause (Shelley and Florence 1961; Weary and Guerrant 1967; Espiritu et al. 1988). The role of candida in urticaria is controversial in the literature. Some studies report on a 70% candida infestation of the general population. In another study with urticaria patients, only 43% were found to be positive, compared to 26% of normal controls. Skin tests with whealing reactions to candida extracts have been noted in 81% of urticaria patients and positive oral provocation tests in 71%. A cessation of urticarial whealing after elimination of intestinal candidosis has been described in 8, or 14, 55, 75 and even 92% of patients in different studies (Möller et al, 1995). Desensitization was successful in 31 to 85%. Some patients with urticaria and intestinal candidosis improve on a diet devoid of sugar, yeast, cheese, chocolate and nonspecific histamine liberators. Taken together, these observations are confusing since in most studies, candida species were not identified and the therapies were highly divergent (Möller et al. 1995). Well conducted studies to resolve this question are still not available. In our own, thoroughly investigated patient group with chronic urticaria (>100 patients), a causative role for candida albicans could not be identified.

The list of parasites causing urticaria is long (Table 2.9). This is most likely due to the well known role of parasites as stimuli of an IgE immune response. Nevertheless, the association of urticaria and parasitic infestation is not unequivocal. In endemic areas, the incidence of urticaria is only increased in children with tolerance induction possibly playing a role in older patients. It is however difficult to explain why the worm burden is not higher in patients with urticaria, compared to controls (Paricha et al. 1972). Furthermore, the urticaria resolves in only 8% of patients with the therapeutic elimination of

Table 2.9. Microorganisms, fungi and parasites as causes of urticaria

Bacteria	Viruses	Parasites	Fungi
Streptococci	Epstein-Barr virus	Giardia lamblia	Candida
Vibrios	Hepatitis B and C virus	Entamoeba histolytica	Trichophyton
Mycoplasma	Coxsackie A 9 virus	Trichomonas hominis	
Pseudomonas	Coxsackie B 5 virus	Plasmodium falciparum	
Helicobacter	ECHO 11 virus	Oxyura, fasciola	
	Herpes virus	Ancylostomata	
	Varicella virus	Strongyloides	
	Measles virus	Onchocerca volvulus	
	Rhinoviruses	Echinococci	
		Schistosomata	
		Trichinella, toxocara	

the worms. This number is only slightly higher (16%) in patients with oxyuriasis (Doeglas 1975).

In Western countries, toxocara and fasciola infestations have been observed as a cause of urticaria. Trichinosis is seen only rarely and manifests itself with periorbital edema, maculopapular rashes, fever and myalgia after ingestion of uncontrolled meat (Wolfrom et al. 1995). Mites are rare causes of urticarial reactions as well (Burns 1986).

Persons traveling in the tropics or subtropics are mainly at risk of developing urticaria due to parasites. The occurrence of urticaria during acute malarial attacks in these patients is well documented. The course of larva migrans through the skin can be recorded well because of linear and polycyclical whealing reactions. Urticarial reactions due to onchocerciasis are easily overlooked because of the lichenified skin of the patients. After penetration of schistosomal larvae through the skin, urticaria, fever, arthralgias, diarrhea and hepatosplenomegaly can develop 4 to 8 weeks later. Rupture of a hydatide liver cyst due to echinococci can cause life threatening anaphylaxis, but antigen linkage due to pressure on the abdomen to cause intermittent whealing. Recently, apparent fish allergies with urticaria have been shown to be due to infestation of the fish with anisakis larvae (Kasuya et al. 1990)

2.5 Internal Diseases

Chronic urticaria is rarely associated with internal diseases (Stafford 1990), with autoimmune and neoplastic processes being most frequent. These include specifically:

- Autoimmune diseases:
  SLE, Still's disease, rheumatic fever, polymyositis;
- Dysproteinemias:
  IgM-paraproteinemia (Schnitzler' syndrome)
  dysproteinemias associated with cold urticaria (see Section 5.4);
- Malignancies:
  Hodgkin's disease, lymphatic leukemia, non-Hodgkin's-lymphomas, polycythemia vera, carcinoma of colon and rectum;
- Diverse other diseases:
  Sarcoidosis,
  Amyloidosis (+ deafness = Muckle-Wells syndrome).

The underlying mechanisms may involve disturbances of the immune system, the expression of neoantigens or the secretion of mediators from transformed cells. The increased frequency of antimicrosomal thyroid antibodies, the recently described anti-IgE and anti-IgE-receptor antibodies in an increased number of patients with chronic urticaria, and the cessation of urticaria after surgical treatment or chemotherapy all fit with this concept (see Section 2.2.1).

Urticaria can precede SLE by up to one year, and it occurs at any time in 4–7% of patients during the course of their disease (Doeglas 1975). Histologically, 90% of patients have an urticarial vasculitis (see Chapter 8). There is no clear correlation between serological findings, the severity of the SLE and the activity of urticaria.

Urticaria can also precede clinical manifestations in Still's disease, lymphoma and leukemia by months or years. 25% of patients with those diseases have an urticaria, while the incidence of urticaria in rheumatic fever is only 1.7% (Czarnetzki 1986). In patients with coeliac disease and associated whealing, institution of a gluten-free diet is associated with remission of the urticaria (Hautekeete et al. 1987).

In the past years, there have been case reports of chronic, only rarely itching urticaria associated with IgM-macroglobulinopathy (Schnitzler's syndrome: Berdy and Bloch 1991; Kropp and Czarnetzki 1994). Associated symptoms of varying intensity are leukocytosis, thrombocytopenia, anemia, increased ESR, bouts of fever, arthralgia, osteomyalgia, lymphadenopathy as well as increased serum fibrinogen and IgG antibodies against IL-1. In these patients, there is often a perivascular neutrophilic infiltrate, but usually neither leukocytoclastic vasculitis nor signs of complement activation. None developed malignant disease over a course of 4 to 9 years. In several other patients with continuous fever and increased ESR, the disease had a fulminant course, with lethal outcome.

Several families have been reported, with members suffering for years from a periodical, generalized urticaria, accompanied by fever and limbpain, progressive hearing loss and inconsistently occuring nephropathy, with at times renal amyloidosis (Muckle Wells syndrome) (Muckle 1979, Throssell et al. 1996).

2.6 Hormones and Hormonal Dysfunctions

Urticaria due to allergic reactions against endogenous hormones is very rare, whereas hormonal medications are a more likely cause.

In thyroid disease, chronic urticaria as well as angioedema can be associated with an autoimmune disease since antimicrosomal antibodies as well as clinical manifestations like vitiligo and pernicious anemia can be present. High serum levels of antithyroid autoantibodies have been noted in 2 to 26% of patients with chronic urticaria, particularly in women, independent of their thyroid status. The incidence in the normal population is 5.6%. In up to 70%

of these patients with antithyroid antibodies, a 2- to 3-month therapy with 200 μg thyroxin induces symptomatic improvement (Leznoff et al. 1983), as also confirmed more recently (Rumbyrt et al. 1995).

In some women, progesterone induces urticaria, eczema or erythema multiforme during the second half of the menstrual cycle. Often, these patients have taken progesterone-containing contraceptives before. This might have possibly induced a sensitization, as can be verified in some patients on skin test (Farah and Shbaklu 1971; Leech anad Kumar 1981), but not in others (Wilkinson et al. 1995). Paradoxically, pregnancy can induce an improvement of symptoms, probably through an induction of tolerance which has also been used successfully in a therapeutic setting (see below). A possible association between progesterone-induced urticaria and an itchy dermatosis with urticarial aspects which typically occurs during the last trimester in 0.38% of pregnancies (PUPP, pruritic urticarial papules and plaques of pregnancy) is not clarified (Lawley et al. 1979).

Next to contraceptives, insulin is the most frequently used hormonal drug. More recently available gene technology products are less allergenic than depot preparations from animal sources or those containing protamine. Swine insulin differs from human preparations by only one amino acid and is therefore less antigenic than bovine insulin. Contaminations during the production of insulin as well as additives and preservatives are further causes of urticarial reactions in insulin-dependent diabetics. Reactions occur more frequently after short therapeutic interruptions and are severe in 10% of cases, requiring a change of the diabetes therapy. About 40% of insulin-dependent patients have positive skin test reactions and low specific serum IgE levels. The development of IgG-antibodies can be suggestive of an insulin resistance (Jegasothy 1980; Chang et al. 1995).

In this context, it should be mentioned that in some women, IgE-mediated anaphylactic reactions are observed against the seminal fluid of their partners. These antibodies have a specificity against a 14–30 kD protein in the prostate fluid so that a vasectomy is of no help (Ohman et al. 1990). Urticaria and angioedema in response to bovine serum albumin have also been reported during artificial dissemination (Wüthrich et al. 1995).

2.7 Neurologic and Psychological Factors

During the past several centuries, an involvement of the nervous system in urticarial reactions has been postulated. This was e.g. supported by an observation during the first half of this century when a patient with hemiparesis and fish allergy developed wheals only on the uninvolved part of the body (Czarnetzki 1986). During the past years, a number of neurotransmitters have been identified as initiators and modulators of mast cell secretion. In clinical practice, one can repeatedly observe patients whose urticaria develops or exacerbates during stress. In several larger studies, psychological factors and stress were identified as primary cause of the urticaria in 11.5% of patients and in 24–51% as aggravating factor. The personality of chronic urticaria patients has been diversely described as unstable, sensitive, cyclothymic, inclined to be tense, anxious and depressive, rigid, introverted and nervous, with frequent psychosomatic complaints (migraine, headaches, chronic gastritis, peptic ulcers) (Rees 1957; Lindemayr et al. 1981).

These findings cannot be upheld using modern tools of psychosomatic testing (Hashiro and Okamura 1994; Badoux and Levy 1994; Hein et al. 1996), and they can mostly be attributed to the vexing symptoms which in turn may be explained by the effects of mast cell mediators, particularly histamine, also on the nervous system.

Earlier reports relating suppression of whealing reactions and tuberculin reactions during hypnosis could not been reproduced in more recent times. Nevertheless, one should not disregard the repeatedly observed prominent placebo effects in urticaria patients. These observations are difficult to differentiate from the normally fluctuating course and the high spontaneous remission rate in urticaria.

2.8 Stinging Insects and Plants

For the sake of completeness, urticarial reactions to stinging insects and plants like nettles should be mentioned at this point. Almost all venoms contain vasoactive amines, even leukotrienes, in addition to histamine liberators (Czarnetzki et al. 1990a + b). This explains the urticarial reactions at sites of stings even in nonallergic persons. In patients with mastocytosis without sensitization, individual insect stings can induce an anaphylactic shock with lethal outcome due to the massive release of mast cell mediators via histamine liberators. Patients with genuine insect venom allergies mostly develop urticarial reactions, flushing and angioedema in addition to their life threatening anaphylactic reactions (Reisman 1994). Some authors have pointed out that urticaria without systemic reactions seems to be a prognostically favorable sign in these patients. Multiple insect stings in children (misleadingly described as papular urticaria) is frequently misdiagnosed as systemically induced acute urticaria.

Literature

Becker CG, Dubin T, Wiedeman HP (1976) Hypersensitivity to tobacco antigen. Proc Natl Acad Sci USA 73:1712-1716

Badoux A, Levy DA (1994) Psychologic symptoms in asthma and chronic urticaria. Ann Allergy 72:229-234

Berdy SS, Bloch K (1991) Schnitzler's syndrome: A broader clinical spectrum J Allergy Clin Immunol 87:849-854

Boch SA (1987) Prospective appraisal of complaints of adverse reaction to foods in children during the fist 3 years of life. Pediactrics 79:683-688

Burns DA (1987) Papular urticaria produced by the mite Listrophorus gibbus. Clin Exp Dermatol 12:200-201

Cardot E, Tillie-Leblond I, Jeannin P, Facon A, Breuil K, Patte F, Tonnel A-B (1995) Anaphylactic reaction to local administration of rifamycin SV. J Allergy Clin Immunol 95:1-7

Chang HH, Leong KP, Loh KC (1995) Primary systemic allergy to human insulin: recurrence of generalized urticaria after successful desensitization. Allergy 50:984-987

Ochinsky S, Chosidow O, Kuentz M, Man N, Fraitag S, Pelisse JM, Revuz J (1991) Cogan's syndrome. An unusual etiology of urticarial vasculitis. Dermatologica 183:218-220

Crespo JF, Pascual C, Dominguez C, Ojeda I, Muñoz FM, Esteban MM (1995) Allergic reactions associated with airborne fish particles in IgE-mediated fish hypersensitive patients. Allergy 50:257-261

Czarnetzki BM (1986) Urticaria. Springer, Berlin

Czarnetzki BM (1989) Urticaria. In: Norris D (ed) Immune mechanisms in cutaneous disease. Dekker, New York, pp 653-670

Czarnetzki BM, Thiele T, Rosenbach R (1990a) Immunoreactive leukotrienes in nettle plants (Urtica urens). Int Arch Allergy appl Immunol 91:43-46

Czarnetzki BM, Thiele T, Rosenbach T (1990b) Evidence for leukotrienes in animal venoms. J Allergy Clin Immunol 85:505-509

Doeglas HNG (1975) Chronic urticaria. Clinical and pathogenetic studies on 141 patients. Dykstra Niemeyer, Groningen

Espiritu BR, Szpindor-Watson A, Zeitz HJ, Thomas LL (1988) IgE-mediated sensitivity to Trichophyton rubrum in a patient with chronic dermatophytosis and Cushing's syndrome. J Allergy Clin Immunol 81:847-851

Farah FS, Shbaklu Z (1971) Autoimmune progesterone urticaria. J. Allergy Clin Immunol 48:257-261

Finke SR, Grieco MH, Connell JT, Smith ED, Sherman WB (1965) Results of comparative skin tests with penicilloylpolylysine and penicillin in patients with penicillin allergy. Am J Med 38:71-82

Friedmann D, Picard-Dahan C, Grossin M, Belaïch S (1995) Chronic urticaria revealing an HIV infection. Eur J Dermatol 5:40-41

Grabbe J, Haas N, Czarnetzki BM (1994) Die Mastzelle. Hautarzt 45:55-64

Hashiro M, Okumura M (1994) Anxiety, depression, psychosomatic symptoms and autonomic nervous function in patients with chronic urticaria. J Dermatol Sci 8:129-135

Hautekeete ML, DeClerck LS, Stevens WJ (1987) Chronic urticaria associated with coeliac disease. Lancet I:157

Hein UR, Czarnetzki BM, Haustein U, Seikowski K, Aberer W, Rufli T, Klapp BF (1996) Zur Beziehung zwischen chronischer Urtikaria und larvierter Depression/Somatisierungsstörung. Hautarzt 47:20-23

Hide M, Francis DM, Grattan CEH, Hakimi J, Kochan JP, Greaves MW (1993) Autoantibodies against the high-afinity IgE receptor as a cause of histamine release in chronic urticaria. N Engl J Med 328:1599-1604

Jegasothy BV (1989) Allergic reactions to insulin. Int J Dermatol 84:227–237
Kanazawa K, Yaoita H, Tsuda F, Okamoto H (1996) Hepatitis C virus infection in patients with urticaria. J Am Acad Dermatol 35:195–198
Kasuya S, Hamano H, Izumi S (1990) Mackerel-induced urticaria and Anisakis. Lancet 335: 665
Kropp JD, Czarnetzki BM (1994) Urtikaria Vaskulitis und Schnitzler-Syndrom. Allergologie 17:17–20
Lawley TJ, Hertz KC, Wade TR, Ackerman AB, Katz SI (1979) Pruritic urticarial papules and plaques of pregnancy. JAMA 241:1696–1699
Leech SH, Kumar P (1981) Cyclic urticaria. Ann Allergy 46:201–203
Leznoff A, Josse RG, Denburg J, Dolovich J (1983) Association of chronic urticaria and angioedema with thyroid autoimmunity. Arch Dermatol 119:636–640
Liebermann P (1991) Anaphylactoid reactions to radiocontrast material. Annals Allergy 67:91–100
Lin RY (1992) A perspective on penicillin allergy. Arch Int Med 152:930–937
Lindemayr H, Gathmann P, Cermak T, Grunberger J (1981) Ist die chronische Urticaria eine psychosomatische Erkrankung? Z Hautkr 56:28–40
McGowen EM (1966) Menthol urticaria. Arch Dermatol 94:62–63
McGrath KG, Zeffren B, Alexander J, Kaplan K Patterson R (1985) Allergic reactions to streptokinase consistent with anaphylactic or antigen-antibody complex-mediated damage. J Allergy Clin Immunol 76:453–457
Möller A, Zuberbier T, Chantraine-Hess S, Czarnetzki BM (1995) Bedeutung der Fokussuche für die Urtikaria-Diagnostik. Allergologie 11:547–552
Muckle TJ (1979) The "Muckle-Wells" syndrome. Br J Dermatol 100:87–92
Odeh M, Oliven A (1992) Urticaria and angioedema induced by low-molecular-weight heparin. Lancet 340:972–973
Ohman JL, Malkiel S, Lewis S, Lorusso JR (1990) Allergy to human seminal fluid: Characterization of the allergen and experience with immunotherapy. J Allergy Clin Immunol 85:103–107
Olson S, Esterly N (1990) Urticaria and Lyme disease. J Am Acad Dermatol 22:1114–1116
Ormerod AD, Reid TMS, Main RA (1987) Penicillin in milk – its importance in urticaria. Clin Allergy 17:229–234
Rappaport BZ, Hoffman MM (1941) Urticaria due to aliphatic aldehydes. JAMA 116: 2656–2659
Reisman RE (1994) Insect stings. New Engl J Med 331:523–527
Rees L (1957) An aetiological study of chronic urticaria and angioneurotic oedema. J Psychosom Res 2:172–189
Rumbyrt JS, Katz JL, Schocket AL (1995) Resolution of chronic urticaria in patients with thyroid autoimmunity. J Allergy Clin Immunol 96:901–905
Sampson HA, Metcalfe DD (1992) Food allergies. JAMA 268:840–844
Saxon A, Adelman DC, Patel A, Hajdu R, Calandra GB (1988) J Allergy Clin Immunol 82:213–217
Schlumberger HD (1983) Pseudoallergic reactions to drugs and chemicals. Ann Allergy 51:317–324
Schlumberger HD, Löbecke EA, Kallos P (1974) Acetylic acid intolerance. Lack of N-acetylsalicylic acid species specific antibodies in the serum of intolerant individuals. Acta Med Scand 196:451–458
Shelley WB, Florence R (1961) Chronic urticaria due to mold hypersensitivity. A study in cross sensitization and autoerythrocyte sensitization. Arch Dermatol 83:549–558
Speer F, Casas Carrasco L, Kimura CC (1978) The management of urticaria. Ann Allergy 40:387–392

Stafford CT (1990) Urticaria as a sign of systemic disease. Ann Allergy 64:264-270
Sutton BJ, Gould HJ (1993) The human IgE network. Nature 366:421-428
Tebbe B, Geilen CC, Schulzke J-D, Bojarski C, Radenhausen M, Orfanos CE (1996) Helicobacter pylori infection and chronic urticaria. J Am Acad Dermatol 34:685-686
Throssell D, Feehally J, Trembath R, Walls J (1996) Urticaria, arthralgia, and nephropathy without amyloidosis: another variant of the Muckle-Wells syndrome? Clin Genet 49: 130-133
Vaida GA, Goldman MA, Bloch KJ (1983) Testing for hepatitis B virus in patients with chronic urticaria and angioedema. J Allergy Clin Immunol 72:193-198
Wantke F, Hemmer W, Haglmüller T, Götz M, Jarisch R (1995) Anaphylaxis after dental treatment with a formaldehyde-containing tooth-filling material. Allergy 50:274-276
Warin RP, Champion RH (1974) Urticaria. Saunders, London
Weary PE, Guerrant JL (1967) Chronic urticaria in association with dermatophytosis. Arch Dermatol 95:400-401
Wilkinson SM, Beck MH, Kingston TP (1995) Progesterone-induced urticaria - need it be autoimmune? Brit J Dermatol 133:792-794
Wolfrom E, Chêne G, Boisseau H, Beylot C, Géniaux M, Taïeb A (1995) Chronic urticaria and Toxocara canis. Lancet 345:196
Wüthrich B (1988) IgE-mediated food intolerance. J Allergy Clin Immunol 81:495-504
Wüthrich B (1983) Allergische und pseudoallergische Reaktionen der Haut durch Arzneimittel und Lebensmitteladditiva. Schweiz Rundschau Med (PRAXIS) 72:691-699
Wüthrich B, Stern A, Johansson SGO (1995) Severe anaphylactic reaction to bovine serum albumin at the first attempt of artificial insemination. Allergy 50:179-183
Wüthrich B, Bianchi-Kusch E, Johansson SGO (1996) Allergic urticaria and angioedema caused by a hemostatic sponge of bovine fibrin used in tooth extraction. Allergy 51: 49-51
Zuberbier T, Chantraine-Heß S, Czarnetzki BM (1995) The role of food intolerance in chronic urticaria - a prospective study. Acta Derm Venereol (Stockh) 75:484-487
Zuberbier T, Czarnetzki BM (1992, 1993) Nahrungsmittelunverträglichkeit, I und II. Hautarzt 43:805-911, 44:57-62
Zuberbier T, Iffländer J, Semmler C, Czarnetzki BM (1996) Acute urticaria - clinical aspects and therapeutic responsiveness. Acta Derm Venereol (Stockh) 76:295-297

3 Acute and Chronic Urticaria

T. ZUBERBIER and B.M. HENZ

3.1 Definition

These two types of urticaria are only distinguished on the basis of disease duration. By definition, acute urticaria lasts maximally 6 weeks (some authors use four weeks as the cut-off line), but can reoccur intermittently in weeks or months. Chronic urticaria is defined as lasting longer than 6 weeks, with either a continuous or a recurrent pattern, depending on the frequency of the urticarial bouts (see Table 1.2). By convention, the term chronic urticaria is restricted to systemically induced urticaria, in contrast to chronic types of urticaria that are induced by physical causes and those due to mast cell proliferation (mastocytosis). Cholinergic urticaria and urticarial vasculitis are generally not grouped with chronic urticaria because of their distinct pathogenesis and clinical aspect (see Chapters 6 and 8).

3.2 General Aspects

Acute and chronic urticaria have already been discussed in the two preceding chapters, and details regarding diagnostic and therapeutic procedures are given in Chapters 10 and 11. Since both types of urticaria are particularly frequent in daily clinical practice, this chapter summarizes briefly their most important aspects.

3.3 Epidemiology

There are no reliable data regarding the incidence of chronic urticaria in the literature. Well known data are summarized in Section 1.4. The prevalence within the general population is probably below 0.5 %, with an average disease duration of several years.

Acute urticaria is far more frequent, with 12–15% of the population experiencing bouts of the disease at some time during their life (Sheldon et al. 1954). In an earlier study from Virginia, the numbers were even higher (23.5%; Swinny 1941).

3.4 Acute Urticaria

3.4.1 Clinical and Diagnostic Aspects

Acute urticaria is characterized by scattered wheals measuring more than 1 cm and rarely only 2–3 mm in diameter, with surrounding erythema and associated itching. Angioedema can be prominent in some patients. In about 15% of patients, systemic reactions with nausea and moderate dyspnea may be associated.

There is so far little information regarding the clinical course and the therapeutic response in acute urticaria. Patients often report on associated upper airway infection or drug intake. Type I allergic reactions to food seem far less important during adult life than previously assumed (Wüthrich and Häcki-Herrmann 1980; Aoki et al 1994). Thus, in a recent prospective study of 109 patients by Zuberbier et al. (1996), 39.5% of patients with acute urticaria had an associated upper airway infection. The prevalence of atopy was similar to that in the normal population (22%), and type I allergies to food could not be found in any of the patients. In early infancy on the other hand, food intolerance, particularly to cow's milk, is an important factor (Legrain et al. 1990), whereas infections play only a minor role.

In both studies mentioned (Zuberbier et al. 1996; Legrain et al. 1990), a possible association with pseudoallergic reactions to analgesics like aspirin and to sulfonamides was noted (9% with Zuberbier et al. 1996). The relevance of these drugs compared to the associated upper airway infections remains however unclear.

Although it is a generally held belief that the cause of acute urticaria is mostly apparent, we found in a propective study that, despite a careful history and extensive diagnostic tests, the cause of acute urticaria could not be ascertained in most patients with acute urticaria (Zuberbier et al. 1996). Furthermore, none of these 109 patients developed chronic urticaria, whereas the reviews in the literature mostly mention a progression from acute to chronic urticaria in 10% of patients (Czarnetzki 1986). For these reasons, extensive diagnostic procedures in acute urticaria are only justified when a potential life threatening type I allergy is suspected. With regard to pseudoallergic reactions to drugs, it should be kept in mind that about 50% of pseudoallergic reactions to e.g. aspirin develop only after a latency of 6 to 24 hours (Juhlin 1981).

3.4.2
Therapy

The primary goal of therapy, as in all types of urticaria, is the avoidance of elicitors if these are suspected or if they can be identified. During the period of diagnosis, patients should be treated symptomatically. While antihistamines are the mainstay of symptomatic treatment of acute urticaria, corticosteroids may also be instituted in otherwise healthy patients because of the generally transient nature of the disease and since the response is more effective. In a recent study comparing loratadine vs prednisolone in patients with acute urticaria, both agents were equally effective in controlling itching and whealing, but prednisolone was clearly superior regarding time to healing (94% remission within 3 days with 50 mg prednisolone/day vs 66% with 10 mg loratadine/day) (Zuberbier et al. 1996). Patients who failed to clear after 3 days on prednisolone responded to further treatment with loratadine. After at the most 21 days, none of the patients needed further treatment. The fact that no case progressed to chronic urticaria was observed may also be due to the additional antiinflammatory effect of both loratadine and the corticosteroid (see Chapter 11).

3.5
Chronic Urticaria

3.5.1
Clinical Aspects and Diagnosis

Except for the duration of disease, there are no differences between acute and chronic urticaria with regard to the clinical appearance. Angioedema can occur with or without associated whealing.

Chronic urticaria is said to remit according to one source in about 50% of cases within 1 year, with 20% of patients continuing to have symptoms for more than 20 years (Kennard 1995). In another retrospective study, only 32% of 86 patients with chronic urticaria resolved within 3 years (Quaranta et al. 1989).

The numerous possible elicitors of chronic urticaria have been discussed extensively in Chapter 2, although the importance of individual factors is still unclear. Data in the literature are difficult to interpret since most studies were either done retrospectively or on selected patients. In older, larger studies, the percentage of patients with an identified cause is about 25% (Champion et al. 1969, Green et al. 1965). In a more recent retrospective analysis, the number was even less than 10% (Quaranta et al. 1989). More recent prospective studies employing dietary treatment paint a far more optimistic picture. Thus, Haustein (1996) noted improvement in 29% and remission in 44% of chronic urticaria patients treated with a pseudoallergen-free diet after a 6 months follow-up. The numbers were 33% and 25% respectively in patients followed without a dietary treatment during that same time period.

The importance of pseudoallergic reactions in chronic urticaria have already been demonstrated with several other older studies (Juhlin 1980; 1981; Rudzki et al. 1980), but have been criticized for being nonblinded or retrospective.

In a prospective study conducted by us on 67 inpatients with chronic continuous urticaria (Zuberbier et al. 1995), 70% went into remission or clearly improved after a two week low-pseudoallergen diet (for details on the diet, see Appendix D). The causative role of the diet could be proven on double-blind reexposure to a pseudoallergen-rich diet. It should however be emphasized that the role of pseudoallergic reactions to food is discussed controversially. Many physicians feel that only a minority of patients respond to dietary measures. This discrepancy can probably be explained by differences in patient selection and dietary measures employed. The good results of a low-pseudoallergen diet reported by us are only seen in patients with chronic urticaria with daily spontaneous whealing. Dermographic urticaria which by some authors is also summarized under the term chronic urticaria, as well as chronic intermittant urticaria only rarely respond to diet. The second reason for a possible discrepancy is the selection of the diet. The diet employed by us is very strict not only omitting artificial additives but also all fruits and a number of vegetables. This is of major importance since we have now been able to show that a number of naturally occurring aromatic compounds are potent elicitors of pseudoallergic reactions (Pfrommer et al. 1996).

Last but not least success of dietary measures can only be correctly evaluated if they are strictly adhered to for at least 2 weeks. On an outpatient basis, the rate of unwilling mistakes is high unless the possible pitfalls are explained in detail (see Section 11.2.2.1).

Among the remaining non-diet-responsive patients (Zuberbier et al. 1995), 11% improved after treatment of chronic inflammatory processes or infections of the gastrointestinal tract. This held particularly for patients with Helicobacter pylori. Several other recent studies confirm the potential importance of helicobacter-gastritis as a cause of chronic urticaria (Kolibasova et al. 1988; Rebora et al. 1990; Tebbe et al. 1995). The mechanisms involved, e.g. allergens against bacterial proteins versus pseudoallergic reactions to bacteria or products of the inflammatory process, are uncertain. The same holds for intestinal candidosis. In our patients, 16% had markedly positive stools, but no improvement of urticaria was noted after appropriate treatment. Nevertheless, remissions have been reported before in the literature (for review, see Möller et al. 1995). Except for Helicobacter pylori, chronic infections play only a minor role on the basis of our own observations and those reported in the literature (Möller et al. 1995). In contrast to the older literature, type I hypersensitivity is rare in chronic urticaria (Zuberbier et al. 1995).

On the basis of these findings, diagnostic tests should be kept at a minimum in chronic urticaria, unless a specific eliciting agent is suspected. The diagnostic procedures, as done at the clinic in Berlin, are detailed in Chapter 10.

3.5.2 Therapy

As with all types of urticaria, removal of the eliciting agent is the ideal treatment. This is possible in patients with pseudoallergies to food as well as with inflammatory diseases of the gastrointestinal tract. Guidelines for a low-pseudoallergen diet are detailed in Section 11.2.2. The therapy of gastrointestinal causes depends on the specific underlying disease. In case of an infection with helicobacter, the recommended therapy should be adapted to the symptoms, in consultation with a gastroenterologist.

When no specific causal treatment is possible, symptomatic therapy should be instituted, with antihistamines remaining the mainstay of therapy. In the rare H_1-unresponsive patient, a number of possible alternatives are available (see details in Chapter 11).

Literature

Aoki T, Kojima M, Horiko T (1994) Acute urticaria: history and natural course of 50 patients. J Dermatol 21:73-77

Champion RH, Roberts SO, Carpenter RC (1969) Urticaria and angioedema: A review of 554 patients. Br. J Dermatol 81:588-597

Czarnetzki BM (1986) Urticaria. Springer Berlin

Green GR, Koelsche GL, Kierlund RR (1965) Etiology and pathogenesis of chronic urticaria. Ann Allergy 23:30-36

Haustein U (1996) Pseudoallergen-free diet in the treatment of chronic urticaria. Acta Derm Venereol (Stockh) 76:498-499

Kennard CD (1995) Evaluation and treatment of urticaria. Immunol Allergy Clin N Am 15: 785-801

Juhlin L (1980) Incidence of intolerances to food additives. Int J Dermatol 19:548-551

Juhlin L (1981) Recurrent urticaria: clinical investigation of 330 patients. Br J Dermatol 104:369-381

Kolibasova K, Cervenkova D, Hegyi E, Lengyelova J, Toth J (1988) Helicobacter pylori - ein möglicher ätiologischer Faktor der chronischen Urtikaria. Dermatosen 42:235-236

Legrain V, Taieb A, Sage T, Maleville J (1990) Urticaria in infants: a study in 40 patients. Pediatr Dermatol 7:101-107

Möller A, Zuberbier T, Chantraine-Hess S, Czarnetzki BM (1995) Bedeutung der Fokussuche für die Urtikaria-Diagnostik. Allergologie 18:547-552

Pfrommer C, Bastl R, Vieths S, Ehlers I, Henz BM, Zuberbiert T (1996) Characterization of naturally occurring pseudoallergens causing chronic urticaria. J Allergy Clin Immunol 97:367

Rebora A, Drago F, Parodi A (1995) May Helicobacter pylori be important for dermatologists? Dermatology 191:6-8

Rudzki E, Czubalski K, Grzywa Z (1980) Detection of urticaria with food additive intolerance by means of diet. Dermatologia 161:57-62

Sheldon JM, Methews KP, Lovell RG (1954) The vexing urticaria problem. Present concepts of etiology and management. J Allergy 25:525-560

Swinny B (1941) The atopic factor in urticaria. South Med J 34:855-858

Wüthrich B, Häcki-Herrmann D (1980) Zur Ätiologie der Urtikaria. Eine retrospektive Studie anhand von 316 konsekutiven Fällen. Z Hautkr 55:102-111

Tebbe B, Geilen CC, Schulzke JD, Bojarski C, Radenhausen M, Orfanos CE (1996) Helicobacter pylori infection and chronic urticaria. J Am Acad Dermatol 34:685-686

Zuberbier T, Iffländer J, Semmler C, Czarnetzki BM (1996) Acute urticaria - clinical aspects and therapeutic responsiveness. Acta Derm Venereol (Stockh) 76:295-297

Zuberbier T, Chantraine-Hess S, Hartmann K, Czarnetzki BM (1995) The role of food intolerance in chronic urticaria - a prospective study. Acta Derm Venereol (Stockh) 75: 484-487

4 Angioedema

P. MÖLLER and B. M. HENZ

4.1 Definition

Angioedema (synonyms: Quincke-edema, angioneurotic edema) is characterized by the sudden eruption of localized edema of the lower dermis, the subcutis or the submucosal tissue which persists for up to 72 hours. It can occur alone or in association with urticaria and involve individual or several regions of the body, preferentially in a unilateral distribution. Involvement of the upper airways can lead to life threatening situations.

Angioedema can be elicited by diverse causes and pathomechanisms. In a simplified classification, one can distinguish between genetically induced and acquired angioedemas:

I. Acquired angioedema:
   1. Allergic causes
   2. Pseudoallergic causes
   3. Histamine liberators
   4. Physical stimulation
   5. ACE inhibitors
   6. Immune complex diseases (urticarial vasculitis, serum sickness, SLE)
   7. Lymphoproliferative diseases with normal C1-INH
   8. Acquired C1-INH deficiency
      - Type I: lymphoproliferative diseases or other systemic diseases
      - Type II: idiotype-anti-idiotype complexes with increased C1-INH consumption
      - Type III: anti-C1-INH antibodies
   9. Episodic angioedema with hypereosinophilia
   10. Carboxypeptidase-N deficiency
   11. C3b-inactivator deficiency
   12. Systemic capillary leak syndrome
   13. Idiopathic angioedema

II. Familial angioedema
   1. Hereditary angioedema
      - Type I: defective C1-INH-synthesis
      - Type II: inactive C1-INH
      - Type III: protein-bound C1-INH
   2. Familial vibratory angioedema

More than 90% of all chronic angioedemas are idiopathic, and hereditary angioedemas make up less than 1% of all angioedemas. This autosomal dominant defect can be classified into three well defined hereditary C1-inhibitor deficiency types. Type I is most frequent (about 85%) and is due to a quantitative deficit, while the other two types are associated with functional deficiencies. Only a few patients with familial vibratory angioedema have been reported. The majority of acquired angioedema occurs in association with different types of urticaria. Recurrent angioedema with hypereosinophilia (Gleich's syndrome) is very rare and is associated with blood and tissue eosinophilia, urticaria, fever, leukocytosis and autoantibodies against endothelial cells. Severe angioedema, often associated with urticaria, has also been described after treatment with ACE-inhibitors and may be due to a decreased metabolism of bradykinin. As with hereditary C1-inhibitor deficiency, angioedema can also occur on the basis of an acquired C1-inhibitor deficiency. This rare type of angioedema can be further classified into three types: Type I is associated with lymphoproliferative and other systemic diseases, type II is due to idiotype-anti-idiotype complexes, produced by IgG antibodies directed against the idiotype of a monoclonal circulating immunoglobulin, with resulting C1-INH consumption, and in type III, antibodies have been formed against the C1-INH (Ochonsky et al. 1993; Böhler and Wienert 1995).

4.2 Epidemiology

Angioedema occurs at about equal frequency in both sexes. The age incidence ranges from infancy to old age, with the highest frequency of acquired angioedema in the third decade. For hereditary angioedema, the peak incidence of first manifestations is in the first and second decade.

4.3 Clinical Manifestations

4.3.1 Cutaneous Symptoms

In contrast to urticaria, angioedema develops in deeper layers of the skin. The lesions are markedly raised, tend to be pale rather than erythematous, and generally cause pain due to tension rather than itching. They can be solitary or multiple, and recurrences tend to appear at the same sites of predilection. Frequent localizations are the lips, eyelids, tongue, hands, feet, pharynx and genitals. ACE-INH-induced angioedema has a special predilution for the tongue, followed by oropharyngeal involvement (Roberts and Wuerz 1991, Sabroe and Kobza-Black 1997). Lesions appear suddenly and resolve entirely within 24–72 hours. Prodromes of paresthesia and local tension can precede their appearance.

Angioedema mostly occurs simultaneously or alternating with attacks of urticaria. In contrast, the more rare types of hereditary angioedema as well as acquired angioedema due to C1-inhibitor deficiency have no associated whealing. Similarly, associated urticaria is extremely rare (0.3% incidence) in ACE-INH-induced angioedema. Furthermore, the distribution of angioedema lesions is generally unilateral, and stress or trauma are often reported as eliciting causes of hereditary angioedema (Fig. 4.1). Prodromes like itching, warmth or erythema marginatum-like lesions can precede the development of angioedema. Otherwise, the lesions of hereditary angioedema are identical to those of angioedema due to other causes, although important differences exist regarding extracutaneous involvement (see below). ACE-inhibitor-induced angioedema may occur already after the first week of drug intake, although lesions have also been observed for the first time one year after start of treatment. Bilateral periorbital edema may also occur in association with food intake and a rise in body core temperature (Zuberbier et al. 1993)

4.3.2 Extracutaneous Symptoms

Involvement of organs other than the skin is rare in most types of angioedema, although it is frequent and characteristic for hereditary angioedema and angioedema due to acquired C1-INH deficiency. In these patients, angioedema can present as or be associated with abdominal symptoms as well as swellings of the oral cavity and the pharynx, often due to injury e.g. during dental treatment. Laryngeal edema is less frequent but particularly dangerous because of the potentially lethal outcome due to asphyxia. The latter can also

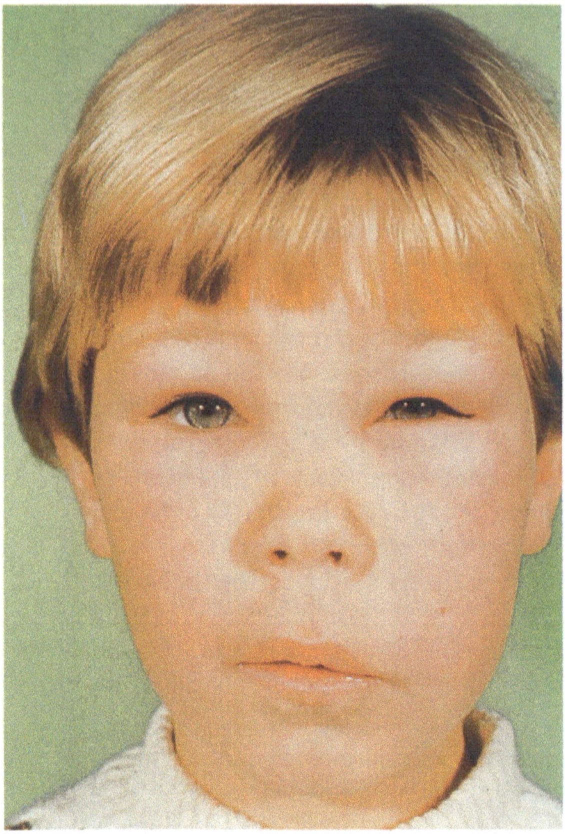

Fig. 4.1. Diffuse unilateral facial edema with pallor in a boy with hereditary angioedema after physical trauma

Table 4.1. Possible extracutaneous symptoms during angioedema

Localization	Symptoms
Oral cavity	Dysphagia, speech disorders
Nasopharynx	Rhinorrhea
Esophagus	Dysphagia
Pharynx	Dysphagia, hoarseness
Larynx	Stridor, dysphagia, speech disorders
Gastrointestinal tract	Abdominal pain, diarrhea, vomiting
Pleural cavity	Cough, pleural pain
CNS	Seizures, hemiparesis, aphasia, headache
Optic nerve	Amaurosis, papillary edema
Urinary bladder	Hematuria

occur due to ACE-INH-induced angioedema. Angioedema in association with urticaria can have similar extracutaneous symptoms as with the particular type of urticaria. Some important extracutaneous symptoms in association with angioedema are summarized in Table 4.1.

4.4 Course and Prognosis

The course of angioedema in association with urticaria is similar to that of acute and chronic urticaria. Hereditary angioedema is generally mild during early childhood, aggravates in late childhood and adolescence and generally improves again with increasing age. In some cases, improvement has already been observed during puberty, and in other cases, patients had their first manifestation only during the fifth and sixth decade. In some patients, an increased incidence of angioedema has been observed during treatment with contraceptives of the estrogen/progesterone type, during menstruation, at the beginning of pregnancy, and after delivery. An improvement of symptoms was observed in some patients after menopause and during the last 6 months of pregnancy. Treatment of an underlying disease induces improvement of symptoms in the majority of patients with acquired C1-INH deficiency with associated angioedema, although this is not invariably so. Episodic angioedema with hypereosinophilia generally has a mild course, lasting over a few years.

4.5 Diagnosis

The diagnosis of angioedema in association with urticaria is the same as that of the concomitant urticaria. For clinical pictures presenting with angioedema only, the rare hereditary angioedema or even rarer acquired C1-INH deficiency-associated angioedema has to be ruled out. Hereditary angioedema is diagnosed on the basis of the clinical characteristics, the positive family history, the lack of urticaria lesions, the typical cutaneous and extracutaneous symptoms (see Section 4.3), radiological and sonographic signs of intestinal edema, the extended duration of lesions and their lack of response to H1-blockers. In acquired C1-INH-deficiency, there is in contrast no positive family history and the symptoms generally begin only in adult life. When hereditary or acquired C1-INH-deficiency associated angioedema is suspected, serum levels of C1-INH, C3 and C4 should be determined (see also Table 4.2). When the C4-level is decreased and the C1-INH and C3-levels are normal, a functional test for C1-INH should be ordered and the C1q-level should be measured as well, in order to exclude the rarer variant of angioedema with

Table 4.2. Complement and C1-INH changes in angioedema (C1-INH changes are generally detectable also in disease-free intervals) n = normal

Plasma levels					Diagnosis
C1-INH (functional test)	C1-INH (immunochemical test)	C1q	C4	C3	
↓	↓		↓		Hereditary angioedema type I
↓	n/↑	n	↓	n	Type II, type III
↓	n/↓	↓	↓	n	Acquired angioedema

functional defects (hereditary or acquired). Patients with acquired C1-INH-deficiency should be screened for possible tumors. Type III acquired angioedema can be diagnosed by an autoantibody against C1-INH (Cicardi 1993) which is important because of the different prognosis and therapeutic responsiveness. Idiopathic angioedema is generally easily distinguished from hereditary angioedema since the first is associated with urticarial lesions and has almost invariably normal complement levels. Other types of angioedema can be identified because of specific eliciting stimuli (physical urticaria, particularly delayed pressure urticaria, drug-induced angioedema) or associated diseases (urticaria pigmentosa, parasitosis, immune complex diseases, lymphomas).

4.6 Differential Diagnosis

Superficially, a number of diseases can be mistaken for angioedema (Table 4.3) (Cooper 1991). Differentiation is however easy when a good history is taken and after a thorough clinical examination. Edemas due to erysipelas are associated with redness, pain and mostly fever, the lesions persist longer, and they respond well to penicillin.

Table 4.3. Differential diagnosis of angioedema

Erysipelas
Contact dermatitis
Photodermatitis
Melkerson-Rosenthal syndrome
Ascher syndrome
Phaeochromocytoma
Tissue edema due to
a) Lymphatic obstruction
b) Cardiac or renal insufficiency
c) Capillary leak syndrome

In Melkerson-Rosenthal syndrome, the recurrent facial edemas generally persist for longer periods and lateron develop granulomatous thickenings. Further possible associated symptoms are a lingua plicata and facial paresis. The rare Ascher syndrome, presenting as edema of the lips and recurrent episodes of eyelid edema, with resulting atrophic, slack skin, is possibly due to an autosomal dominant inheritance (Sanchez et al. 1993). Phaeochromocytoma can rarely present as recurrent bouts of neck swelling (Böhm et al. 1993).

Acute contact eczema with swelling of the eyelids and the remaining face can be distinguished from other types of angioedema due to epidermal changes like blistering and scaling. Tissue edema due to blockade of the lymphatic drainage, caval obstruction, cardiac or renal insufficiency, or the "capillary leak syndrome" are generally more diffuse, develop more slowly and may shift with changes in positioning of the body. Generally, these conditions can be classified correctly after diagnosis of the underlying disease.

In the past, some patients with hereditary angioedema who suffered from recurrent abdominal pain underwent unnecessarily laparoscopy or appendectomy. Generally, these patients have neither signs of peritoneal irritation nor fever, and their pain disappears within 1–3 days. Rarely, a mild leukocytosis is present. One should, however, also consider a normal surgical emergency in these patients.

4.7
Therapy

The treatment of angioedema must be based on the specific underlying causes. After C1-INH-deficiency or defects have been ruled out, the majority of the remaining types of the disease can be treated as described for urticaria (Chapter 11). For some types of angioedema, particularly for familial vibratory angioedema and episodic angioedema with hypereosinophilia, corticosteroids are the most effective drugs. In case of life threatening non-hereditary laryngeal edema that is unresponsive to antihistamines and corticosteroids, 0.3–0.5 ml of 1mg/ml adrenaline solution should be given once or several times. In patients with ACE-inhibitor induced angioedema, drug treatment should be stopped and never be tried again, even with other type of ACE-inhibitor. Antiallergic medication (antihistamines, corticosteroids, adrenaline) are ineffective or associated with rapid rebound-phenomena. In these patients as well as in those with hereditary angioedema, laryngotomy should promptly be performed as a life-saving measure in case of laryngeal edema (Finley et al. 1992).

Treatment of hereditary angioedema is different dependent on the presence of acute attacks, or whether short-term and long-time prophylaxis is needed (Table 4.4).

Table 4.4. Treatment of angioedema due to hereditary or acquired C1-INH defects or deficiency. EACA = epsilon amino caproic acid

I. Acute attacks	1. Analgetics or narcotics against pain 2. C1-INH (500–1000 units[a] in 10 ml physiological NaCl) slowly i.v.; repeat injections in dependence on the clinical picture 3. In case C1-INH preparations are not available, infusion of 500–2000 ml fresh or fresh frozen plasma 4. If indicated, intubation, tracheotomy or coniotomy Note: Adrenaline, corticosteroids and antihistamines are ineffective.
II. Short-term prophylaxis	1. Danazole (about 600 mg/day) 1–10 days before surgery or 2. EACA (about 6 g/d), 2–3 days before surgery or 3. C1-INH (about 500–100 units[a]) i.v. shortly before surgery
III. Long-time prophylaxis	1. Danazole, starting with 600 mg daily, thereafter reduction to the lowest possible dose (about 200 mg) or 2. Tranexamic acid (2–3 g/d, children: 1.5 g/d) 3. EACA (6 g daily; children: 2 g/d) or 4. C1-INH (500 units[a]), i.v., every 4 to 5 days

[a] 1 unit C1-inhibitor concentrate corresponds to a C1-INH activity in 1 ml fresh citrated plasma.

The therapy of choice for acute attacks is substitution with C1-INH concentrate. Normally, slow intravenous infusion of 500–1000 units in 10 ml physiological saline is sufficient to prevent serious complications. The injection can be repeated, dependent on the clinical picture. 500–2000 ml fresh or fresh frozen plasma can be transfused instead. Disadvantages of the latter are possible viral transmission or an initial worsening of angioedema due to increased availability of C2 and C4. Instruments to free the upper airways mechanically (intubation, tracheotomy, coniotomy) should be readily available. Antiallergic treatment with antihistamines, corticosteroids or adrenaline is ineffective.

Long-time prophylaxis is indicated in patients with frequent and severe attacks,. Modified androgens (danazole, stanozolol), have proven to be most effective (Cicardi 1991). Initial doses should be high (danazole about 600 mg/d, stanozolol about 4–6 mg/d). Because of dose-dependent undesired effects (increase of weight, myalgias, dysmenorrhea, virilisation, hepatic toxicity), a lower maintenance dose (danazole about 200 mg/d, stanozolol about 1–2 mg/d) should be aimed at, based on the control of clinical symptoms. Further dose reductions can be obtained by instituting drug-free intervals (e.g. 5 × 200 mg danazole/week).

Antifibrinolytic therapy (tranexamic acid 2–3 g/d; children: 1.5 g/d) and epsilon amino caproic acid (EACA) 6 g/d, children: 2 g/d) can be used as a less effective treatment alternative, with a different spectrum of side effects. Tranexamic acid is slightly superior to EACA. These agents are preferentially used during pregnancy and for children.

In case of unsatisfactory control of symptoms, intermittent longtime substitution treatment with C1-INH is a more costly alternative. A dose of 500 units every 4–5 days is usually sufficient (Bork and Witzke 1989).

For short-term prophylaxis (e.g. before dental or other surgical procedures), patients can be treated with attenuated androgens (danazole 600 mg/d, 1–10 days before surgery), antifibrinolytics (EACA 6 g/d, 2–3 days before surgery) or C1-INH concentrate (500–1000 units shortly before surgery).

Treatment of angioedema due to acquired C1-INH-deficiency must start with a search for underlying causes and their elimination. The same treatment regimen as with hereditary angioedema can be tried. During acute attacks of angioedema, these patients may need much higher doses of C1-INH-concentrate than those with hereditary angioedema. Many patients with underlying lymphoproliferative diseases have profited from longtime prophylaxis with attenuated androgens.

In contrast, patients with C1-INH-autoantibodies seem to respond better to tranexamic acid or corticosteroids.

Literature

Böhler U, Wienert V (1995) Hereditäres Angioödem: Klinik, Pathophysiologie und Therapie. H+G 70:488–495

Böhm M, Steinmüller T, Czarnetzki BM (1993) Rezidivierende paroxysmale Halsschwellungen als Primärmanifestation eines Phäochromozytoms. Dtsch med Wschr, 118: 1011–1014

Bork K, Witzke G (1989) Long-term prophylaxis with C1-inhibitor (C1-INH) concentrate in patients with recurrent angioedema caused by hereditary and acquired C1-inhibitor deficiency. J Allergy Clin Immunol 83:677–682

Cicardi M (1991) Long-term treatment of hereditary angioedema with attenuated androgens. A survey of a 13-year experience. J Allergy Clin Immunol 87:768–773

Cicardi M, Bisiani G, Cugno M (1993) Autommune C1-inhibitor deficiency: Report of eight patients. Am J Med 95:169–175

Cooper KD (1991) Urticaria and angioedema: Diagnosis and evaluation. J Am Acad Dermatol 25:166–176

Finley CJ, Silverman MA, Nunez AE (1992) Angiotensin-converting enzyme inhibitor-induced angioedema: still unrecognized. Am J Emerg Med 10:550–552

Greaves M, Lawlor F (1991) Angioedema: Manifestations and management. J Am Acad Dermatol 25:155–165

Ochonisky S, Intrator L, Wechsler J, Revuz J, Bagot M (1993) Acquired C1 inhibitor deficiency revealing systemic lupus erythematosus. Dermatology 186:261–263

Roberts JR, Wuerz RC (1991) Clinical characteristics of angiotensin-converting enzyme inhibitor-induced angioedema. Ann Emerg Med 20:555–558

Sabroe RA, Kobza-Black A (1997) Angiotensin-converting enzyme (ACE) inhibitors and angio-edema. Br J Dermatol 136:153–158
Sanchez MR, Lee M, Moy JA, Ostreicher R (1993) Ascher syndrome: A mimicker of acquired angioedema. J Am Acad Dermatol 29:650–651
Zuberbier T, Böhm M, Czarnetzki BM (1993) Food intake in combination with a rise in body temperature: a newly identified cause of angioedema. J All Clin Immunol 171: 205–215

5 Physical Urticaria

B. M. Henz

5.1 General Aspects

5.1.1 Definition and Classification

Physical urticaria is defined as a localized or generalized urticarial reaction of the skin or the mucous membranes to different specific physical stimuli. The reason for the overreaction of the skin to otherwise tolerated physical stimuli remains unexplained. In most cases, mast cell degranulation and in some special types of physical urticaria even IgE-dependent sensitization has been demonstrated. A genetic predisposition or associated diseases can sometimes be identified as underlying causes.

Physical urticaria is classified according to the nature of the eliciting stimulus, i.e. mechanical, thermic or electromagnetic (Fig. 5.1). On this basis, dermographic urticaria, delayed pressure urticaria, and vibratory angioedema belong to the group of mechanically induced physical urticaria. Cold and heat urticaria are induced by thermic stimuli, and solar urticaria by electromagnetic waves. There is one case report each for decompression-associated urticaria and X-ray induced urticaria (reviewed in Czarnetzki 1985, 1986), and we have recently observed a patient who reacted with whealing after argon-laser treatment in the absence of urticarial dermographism (unpublished).

In older publications, two other types of urticaria have been grouped with the physical urticarias. Cholinergic urticaria is provoked during physical exercise in a warm environment, but also during psychic stress alone, so that this type of urticaria can not be classified as an urticaria due to physical stimuli. It is therefore dealt with separately in Chapter 6 of this book, together with exercise-induced anaphylaxis. Aquagenic urticaria is elicited by a chemical rather than a physical stimulus to the skin surface, with the water dissolving probably a water-soluble antigen in the epidermis (Czarnetzki et al. 1986). A classification with physical urticaria seems thus inappropriate, and this topic is discussed instead in Chapter 7 on contact urticaria.

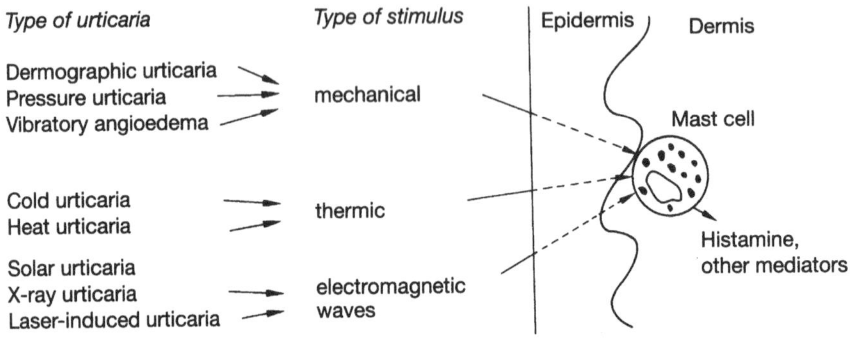

Fig. 5.1. Schematic presentation of different types of urticaria and their respective eliciting stimuli, with resulting release of histamine and other mediators from dermal mast cells

5.1.2
Epidemiology

Up to 50% of all types of chronic forms of urticaria are due to physical urticaria. Its incidence varies depending upon its definition. This holds particularly for urticarial dermographism which is mostly an incidental finding of which patients are unaware, compared to dermographic urticaria where patients present at the physician's office because of an impressive symptomatology. Among physical urticarias, dermographic urticaria is most frequent, even when very strict diagnostic criteria are applied. It is followed in frequency by delayed pressure urticaria, cold urticaria and solar urticaria. Heat contact urticaria and vibratory angioedema are very rare. In cold regions, cold urticaria becomes manifest at a higher frequency.

The most important epidemiologic data on physical urticaria are summarized in Table 5.1. Generally, young adults are more frequently affected. The disease begins mostly without obvious reason, persists over several years, and disappears again spontaneously, although it can also persist for many decades. This holds particularly true for the rare familial types of physical urticaria which are mostly based on an autosomal dominant inheritance.

Familial Types of Physical Urticaria

- Dermographic urticaria
- Familial cold urticaria
- Delayed cold urticaria
- Delayed heat urticaria
- Solar urticaria with erythropoietic protoporphyria
- Vibratory angioedema

Table 5.1. Epidemiologic data on physical urticaria. M = males, F = females, chr = chronic, p = pressure, c = cold, chol = cholinergic, aq = aquagenic, h = heat, s = solar urticaria, d = dermographic urticaria; AE = angioedema, VAE = vibratory angioedema, EIA = exercise induced anaphylaxis, ? = unknown

Urticaria	Mean age at beginning (yrs)	Mean duration (yrs)	M/F	Associated urticaria
Dermographic urticaria	25	6.5	0.4/1.0	chr, p, c, chol, aq, AE
Cold urticaria	18	4.2	0.5/1.0	chr, d, c, aq, VAE, EIA
Pressure urticaria	34	6.0	1.7/1.0	chr, c, h, d
Solar urticaria	28	7.1	0.9/1.0	d, c, h, p
Heat urticaria	37	1.0	0.2/1.0	d, c, s
Vibratory angioedema	?	?	?	d, chol
Familial cold urticaria	Childhood	Life-long	1.7/1.0	

The frequency of atopy is mostly not increased, although other types of urticaria are associated (Table 5.1) and rarely also respiratory or food-related (pseudo-)allergic diseases. Women are more frequently affected than men, except for delayed pressure urticaria and familial cold urticaria.

5.1.3 Clinical Manifestations

The different types of physical urticaria share three common characteristics (Table 5.2): They can be repeatedly elicited by specific stimuli, the symptoms usually develop rapidly, and the lesions disappear rapidly, with the skin again assuming a normal appearance, although the involved area can be refractory to further whealing for a certain time period.

Physical urticaria can be localized, or it can be generalized, with whealing also at distant parts of the skin or involving the entire body surface. Wheals are generally of medium size and irregular, as in ordinary, systemically elicited urticaria, but they tend to be limited to the area of contact, comprising either large or only small circumscribed skin areas, depending on the extent of the eliciting stimulus.

In cold urticaria, one can observe wheals as well as angioedema. Vibratory stimuli generally induce only angioedema. In delayed pressure urticaria, wheals always reach into the deeper dermis and thus resemble angioedema. In familial cold urticaria due to cold wind, the lesions present mostly as a generalized maculopopular rash rather than as urticarial wheals.

Almost all patients with physical urticaria note itching at the site of whealing, although some experience stinging or burning instead. Deep swellings, particularly in areas where the skin can not expand like at the hands and over

Table 5.2. Clinical aspects of physical urticaria

Urticaria	Eliciting stimulus	Time of onset	Duration (hrs)	Diagnostic test
Dermographic urticaria	Firm stroking or scratching	2-5 min	1–3	Firm stroking with the blunt end of a pen or safety pin
Delayed urticarial dermographism	As above	$^1/_2$–8 hrs	1–8	Same as above
Cold urticaria	Cold contact	2-5 min	1–3	Cold objects: ice, cold bath, cold wind or cold air
Delayed pressure urticaria	Static pressure	$^1/_2$–10 hrs	8–72	Locally applied weights
Solar urticaria	UV-light	2–15 min	$^1/_4$–3	Tests with UV-light of different wavelengths
Heat urticaria	Heat contact	2–15 min	$^1/_2$–1	Warm bath
Vibratory angioedema	Vibration	$^1/_2$–1 min	1	Vibrating motor
Familial cold urticaria	Cold wind	$^1/_2$–3 hrs	48	Cold wind and subsequent rewarming

joints, tend to be painful. In some patients, stimuli normally eliciting physical urticaria only cause itching, without recognizable skin changes.

While the majority of wheals in physical urticaria develop rapidly and are of short duration, reactions can also appear with a delay of 2 or even 4–8 hours after stimulation. The most frequent representative of this group is delayed pressure urticaria, with lesions persisting particularly long, namely for up to 3 days.

Depending on the intensity and the extent of stimulation, massive release of histamine and other mast cell mediators occurs, causing systemic symptoms which range from headaches to anaphylactic shock. Involvement of other organs like the lung (shortness of breath) or the intestinal tract (nausea, epigastric pain, diarrhea) are often observed as well. In delayed pressure urticaria and familial cold urticaria, malaise, fever, leukocytosis and arthralgias are often observed.

5.1.4 Diagnosis

In contrast to ordinary acute and chronic urticaria, the diagnosis of physical urticaria is rarely missed because 1. the patient generally recognizes the eliciting stimulus, and 2. the special shape and distribution of wheals or deep edemas allow a correct diagnosis on inspection or by patient history. The diagnosis can be confirmed by elicitation of the wheals, imitating exactly the provoking stimuli in ordinary life.

The methodology of testing for physical urticaria is outlined in Table 5.2 and described below in more detail for each special type of physical urticaria. The results of testing can be documented on a special test sheet (see Appendix C) which can be added to the patient's medical records.

The presence of physical urticaria is easily missed when it coexists with acute or chronic urticaria since the symptomatology of the latter is generally more impressive. In each patient presenting with urticaria or even itching, a test for dermographic urticaria should therefore be done, and a history regarding other types of physical urticaria should be taken as well.

5.1.5 Therapy

As with other types of urticaria, effective treatment of physical urticaria requires an exact diagnosis. Whenever possible, underlying causes must be treated in secondary types of physical urticaria due to other diseases. Furthermore, the patient must be instructed to avoid eliciting stimuli. This is particularly important when symptoms are intense or even life threatening.

Since the majority of symptoms is due to histamine release, antihistamines almost invariably afford relief from itching and suppress whealing reactions. In case of non-responsiveness, other inflammatory agents can be tried. Corticosteroids should be avoided because of the chronicity of the disease. In most types of physical urticaria, a refractory period can be used to induce short-time tolerance.

Details regarding the therapy of special types of physical urticaria are discussed in the subsequent sections.

5.2 Dermographic Urticaria

S. Jeep and B. M. Henz

5.2.1 Definition

Dermographic or facticial urticaria is defined as localized redness, itching and whealing elicited on the skin over the area of stroking with moderate pressure (e.g. with a tongue depressor, the closed end of a ball-point-pen or a safety pin) (Breathnach et al. 1983, Czarnetzki 1986, Wong et al. 1984). As a consequence, whealing reactions will appear that differ regarding latency, size and symptoms, as outlined in Table 5.3. By definition, dermographic urticaria is a rapidly appearing, intensely itching whealing reaction while urticarial dermographism has no associated subjective symptoms at all (Jeep and Czarnetzki 1994).

5.2.2
Epidemiology

Dermographic urticaria is the most frequent type of physical urticaria. It is observed in all age groups, with a peak prevalence in young adults (second to third decade of life) and an overall prevalence of 1.5–5%. Delayed urticarial dermographism and cholinergic urticarial dermographism are in contrast very rare. Data regarding the frequency of urticarial dermographism vary widely (between 1.5–50.0%), depending on the intensity of the eliciting pressure, whether a distinction is made between dermographic urticaria and urticarial dermographism and depending on the type of subjects examined (patients with chronic recurrent urticaria, dermatology or allergy patients, or the normal population).

The higher the pressure during testing, the greater the number of persons who react with urticarial dermographism. Using a standardized dermographometer applying 12.7×10^5 Pa, the authors have recently noted a 44.6% prevalence of urticarial dermographism among 74 test subjects, in accordance with data from other groups (Henz et al. 1996).

Dermographic urticaria as well as urticarial dermographism may disappear within 6 months but can persist for many years (Table 5.1). In the latter case, episodic associated itching can make it difficult to clearly separate the two conditions.

5.2.3
Clinical Aspects

Patients with dermographic urticaria suffer most from the intermittent, generalized pruritus and the chronic recurring whealing reactions, particularly at

Table 5.3. Different types of urticarial dermographism dependent on latency until appearance and duration of the wheal as well as associated symptoms

	Latency (min)	Duration (min)	Itching
Dermographic urticaria	1– 5	20–30	+++
Urticarial dermographism	2– 10	10–30	–
Delayed urticarial dermographism/ dermographic urticaria	30–240	12–48 h	–
Cholinergic urticarial dermographism/ dermographic urticaria	5– 10	20–30	+/–

sites of shearing forces on the skin, e.g. in the belt region and the groin, due to tightly fitting and rubbing pieces of garments such as belts. The patients also report on linear wheals after scratching of the skin. In all patients with urticarial dermographism or dermographic urticaria, it should be kept in mind that increased whealing can also occur during prick testing for type I allergies. Such false positive reactions should be considered in patients reacting to numerous allergens as well as the saline control.

5.2.4 Diagnosis and Differential Diagnosis

There are no specific laboratory tests for dermographic urticaria. The diagnosis is made simply by testing for the presence of dermographism. This is done by applying sheering forces, e.g. via firm linear stroking with a tongue depressor or the closed end of a ballpoint pen over the upper back. The diagnosis is made as follows, depending on the type of reaction:

1. Localized erythema and whealing extending over the area of stroking within seconds to minutes, with associated itching: *dermographic urticaria* (Fig. 5.2)
2. Appearance of localized erythema and whealing not extending over the area of stroking, within 5–10 minutes, without associated itching: *urticarial dermographism*
3. Development of deep, linear, persisting whealing with mild or no erythema, mostly with associated burning or pain, within 1–4 hours after elicitation: *delayed urticarial dermographism/dermographic urticaria*
4. Appearance of localized erythema and multiple pin-point size wheals within 5–10 minutes after stroking: *cholinergic urticarial dermographism* (Fig. 5.3). When this type of reaction is intense, with associated itching and possibly confluent lesions (peau d'orange), it should be designated *cholinergic dermographic urticaria.*

Delayed urticarial dermographism can be associated with ordinary urticarial dermographism, in which case the rapidly developing wheals disappear after 20–30 minutes, to reappear after 1–2 hours at the same sites, with deeper swellings that persist over many hours. The initial reaction can however also be only an erythema, with the whealing reaction occurring only 1–4 hours later. These delayed reactions are easily missed unless they are specifically looked for.

Dermographic urticaria and urticarial dermographism as well as delayed urticarial dermographism must be differentiated from delayed pressure urticaria which is elicited by resting rather than shearing forces. This distinction is important because delayed pressure urticaria differs from dermographic reactions in terms of pathogenesis, clinical manifestation and therapy (see below).

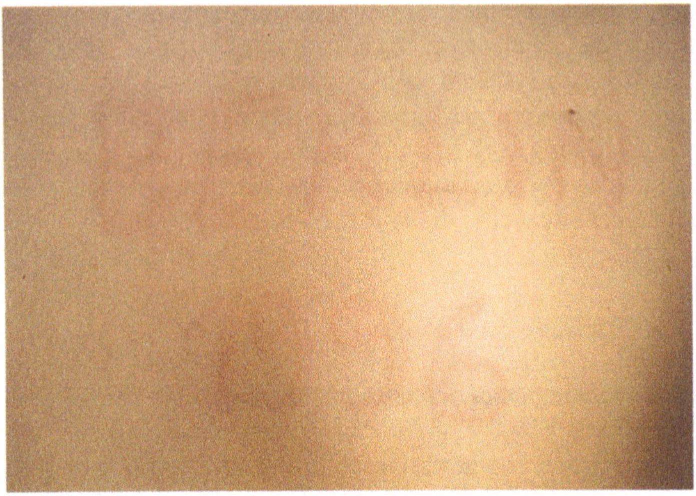

Fig. 5.2. Lesions of dermographic urticaria, with redness and itching appearing 1 minute after application of linear pressure with a dermographometer

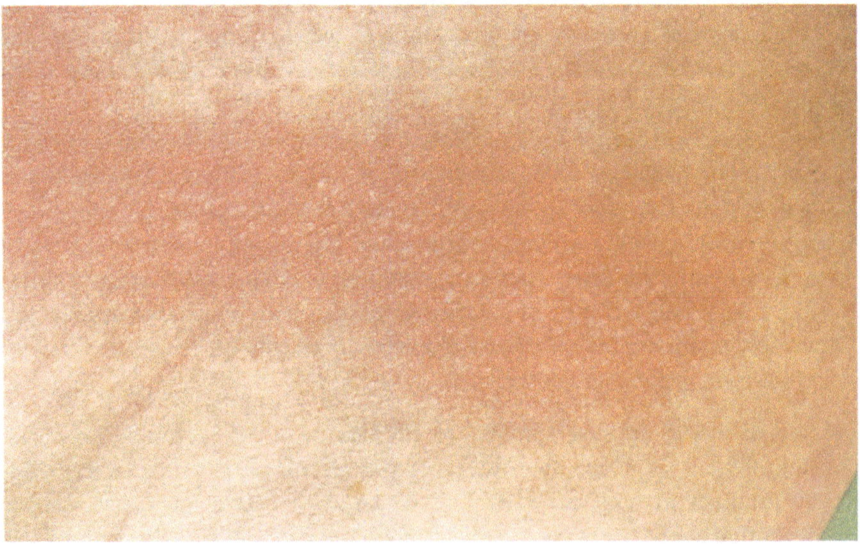

Fig. 5.3. Cholinergic dermographic urticaria in a patient with associated cholinergic urticaria. Instead of the usual linear wheal, pin-point size wheals with surrounding erythema and associated itching have developed in this patient during testing for dermographism

5.2.5
Associated Symptoms and/or Diseases

The causes of dermographic urticaria and urticarial dermographism are largely unknown. Some subjects with simple urticarial dermographism seem to be constitutionally predisposed to these exaggerated reactions. In others, penicillin and other drugs seem to initiate such overreactivity which can then persist for many months after cessation of treatment. Furthermore, the condition seems to occur frequently in association with parasitosis, during pregnancy and at sites of previous contact dermatitis or insect stings, or in tattoos (see Table 5.4).

5.2.6
Therapy

Simple urticarial dermographism generally requires no treatment. With the other types of urticarial dermographism, associated diseases (Table 5.4) must be ruled out or treated. Patients must be instructed to avoid eliciting stimuli like tight clothes, certain drugs (penicillin, aspirin, lidocaine, famotidine), rigorous showering or any stimulus that elicits or activates itching, including stress (Schafer 1995).

Non-sedating antihistamines (H1-blockers like cetirizine, terfenadine, loratadine) generally suffice to control the symptoms (Cap et al. 1985). At night, higher than usual doses of these drugs or the potent sedating H1-blocker hydroxyzine may be used in patients with severe pruritus (Breathnach et al. 1983).

In cooperative patients, a low-pseudoallergen diet (see Appendix D) can be tried for about 4–6 weeks since it occasionally induces remissions, although at a far lower rate than in chronic urticaria (own unpublished results).

Table 5.4. Associated symptoms and/or diseases in dermographic conditions. *UD: urticarial dermographism*

Dermographic urticaria	Simple UD	Delayed UD/ dermographic urticaria	Cholinergic UD/ dermographic urticaria
Acute urticaria	Constitutional	Pressure urticaria	Cholinergic urticaria
Chronic urticaria	After drugs	Chronic urticaria	Aquagenic urticaria
Mastocytosis	Chronic urticaria		
Parasitosis			
Pressure urticaria			

5.3 Delayed Pressure Urticaria

S. Krüger-Krasagakes and B. M. Henz

5.3.1 Definition

Patients with this type of physical urticaria develop typical lesions (see below) particularly at skin areas that are exposed to high pressure, e.g. palms and soles, the buttocks, the upper back and rarely also the face. After application of pressure, wheals or deep painful swellings develop after a latency of 4–8 hours (range 0.5–10 hours) and persist for 30 ± 8 hours (range 8–48 hours). In recent years, the possible existence of immediate type pressure urticaria is also being discussed (wheals within 5–10 minutes after application of static pressure). This entity must be differentiated from dermographic urticaria, with whealing appearing after application of shearing forces.

5.3.2 Epidemiology

The frequency of pressure urticaria among patients with chronic urticaria ranges from 2–35%, depending on the investigator and the method for evaluation (Barlow et al. 1993). Males (65–80%) and persons of young to medium age groups are preferentially affected. The mean age at onset of the disease is about 30 years (range 5–63 years), the mean duration 6–9 years (range 1–40 years). Pressure urticaria becomes particularly evident in patients employed in jobs requiring heavy physical work, and 11% of patients are severely disabled in their daily physical activities (Dover et al. 1988; Sussman et al. 1982; Czarnetzki et al. 1984).

5.3.3 Clinical Manifestations

Local manifestations: The individual lesions in pressure urticaria present as erythematous, deep swellings (Fig. 5.4), at times with a central pallor. The size of the lesions fits exactly the area of application of pressure. Due to the deep swelling, one can accentuate the peau d'orange appearance of the lesion by squeezing the wheal between thumb and index finger (Fig. 5.5). The skin is warm over the site of the swelling. Most patients experience itching before the whealing appears, but some also report pain, burning or stinging. When the swellings involve joints or muscles, the patients often experience marked pain.

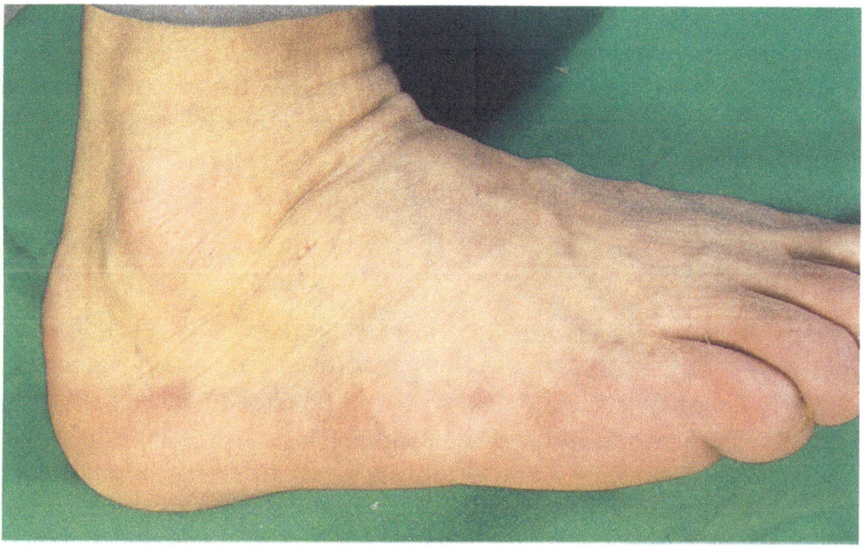

Fig. 5.4. Swelling and redness at pressure sites due to shoes in a patient with delayed pressure urticaria. The soles of the feet were swollen as well

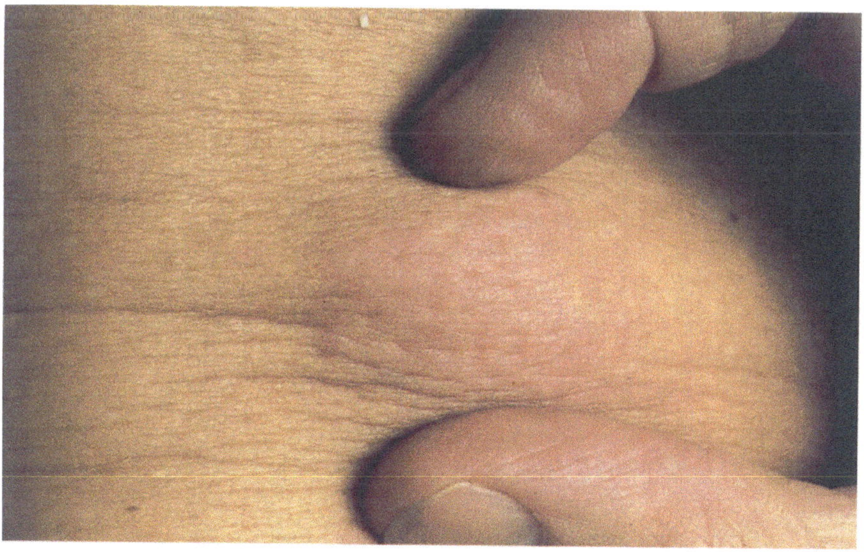

Fig. 5.5. Deep swelling and redness at the site of pressure testing (1800 g, 10 min) on the back of a patient with delayed pressure urticaria. The swelling developed only 6 hours after testing. The typical orange peal phenomenon is evident by application of lateral pressure to the wheal

Systemic manifestations: About 50% of patients with pressure urticaria complain about additional extracutaneous symptoms such as shivering, fever, dizziness, arthralgias, increased perspiration, nausea, headache, shortness of breath or tiredness. Some patients observe a correlation between the intensity of the symptoms and physical or psychic stress.

5.3.4 Associated Diseases

Other types of urticaria have been reported in from 25–94% of patients with pressure urticaria. More than 50% have an associated delayed dermographic urticaria, i.e. patients develop redness and whealing at sites where urticarial dermographism was elicited 2–4 hours earlier (Dover et al. 1988). Whealing of the so-called delayed urticarial dermographism can persist for more than 8 hours. Patients with pressure urticaria have a slightly increased frequency of atopic diseases in their own and the family history. Some investigators also describe an increased number of positive prick test reactions but interpret these as mostly false positive due to associated urticarial dermographism (Czarnetzki et al. 1987). An increased incidence of aspirin intolerance is found by some investigators (Dover et al. 1988).

5.3.5 Diagnosis

The diagnosis of pressure urticaria can be made solely on the basis of a good medical history. Particular attention must be paid to the distribution of the lesions, their time of appearance several hours after application of pressure, and the shape of the wheals. The frequently associated other types of urticaria with a different time course and distribution of the wheals must be considered. Differentiation of the different types of urticaria can only be made by specific questioning in patients who observe themselves well. The presence of the typical deep whealing at the sites of predilection (see Section 5.5.3) and physical examination supports the diagnosis which requires confirmation by reproduction of the lesions. For this purpose, Illig and Kunick (1969) built a special instrument that allows for the application of different weights for variable times on the back of a patient. A simple alternative consists in applying weights from 3–10 kg with a broad belt over the shoulder or the upper thigh, with the patient in a sitting position and perhaps even a glass sphere (marble) placed below the weighted cuff to increase and localize the pressure stimulus (Warin 1987). The weights should remain in place for 10–30 minutes, and possible changes of the skin at the site of application should be recorded immediately after removal of the weights as well as 4, 6, 8 and possibly also

24 hours thereafter. Concomitantly, the patient's back should be scratched with a dermographometer or a similar device in order not to overlook the co-existence of delayed urticarial dermographism.

In case of negative test results in a patient with a positive history, testing should be repeated at different skin areas at 48 hour intervals since patients with proven pressure urticaria fail to have regularly positive test results. In some patients, pressure tests are e.g. only positive on the shoulder but not on the back. Pressure urticaria often also has a fluctuating course which coincides with the activity of a simultaneously existing chronic urticaria (Estes and Young 1981). Thus, the major reasons for false negative pressure tests are:

- a refractory test site because of a recent application of pressure during normal life
- fluctuations in the sensitivity of the skin
- immunosuppressive treatment, e.g. with corticosteroids
- insufficient testing: weights are too low or the time of application is too short

Laboratory findings and histological examinations can add further support to the clinical diagnosis. Most of the changes are however not disease specific. Thus, 70% of all pressure urticaria patients have a mild to moderately raised ESR, and leukocytosis occurs in 20–53%, without correlation to disease activity. Serum enzymes, immunoglobulins, complement levels, C1 INH, α_2-macroglobulin and α_1-antitrypsin are normal. On histology of lesional biopsies, an inflammatory infiltrate consisting of eosinophils, neutrophils, T-lymphocytes and activated macrophages is particularly prominent around appendages in the deep dermis and can also extend into the subcutis. Mast cell numbers are increased, even in normal skin. In contrast to other types of urticaria, there is no expression of the cytokine MIF, and immunoglobulin or complement deposits are not detectable on immunofluorescence (Czarnetzki et al. 1984, 1989). Fibrin deposits have been found by some investigators, but not by others. The histological findings suggest a cell-mediated immune reaction against an as yet unknown antigen.

5.3.6 Differential Diagnosis

The deep swellings of the lesions can mimic erysipelas or angioedema. Superficial, itching urticarial lesions at sites such as the belt region can be part of acute or chronic urticaria. These lesions which were not provoked by pressure can be interpreted as a Köbner-phenomenon.

5.3.7 Therapy

Of all types of urticaria, pressure urticaria is most difficult to treat. Classical oral or intravenous antihistamines are ineffective. An improvement on high doses of cetirizine (>30 mg/d), which was found to be effective in Greek patients (Kontou-Fili et al. 1991) could not be confirmed by us and others (unpublished and personal communication, Prof. Greaves, London). The beneficial effect of cetirizine in Greek patients was atributed to its inhibitory effect on eosinophils.

Corticosteroids induce a reproducible improvement in all patients with pressure urticaria. Because of the chronicity of the disease and the potential adverse effects, this treatment is, however, indicated only in case of serious problems in daily life and at work. A maintenance dose below the Cushing level should be aimed at, with minimal adverse events. Individual local lesions can also be reduced in size by the application of potent topical steroids.

Dapsone, at a dose of 50–100 mg/d, can totally control symptoms in some patients and is worth a trial. Lesions reappear however after cessation of treatment. Sulfazalazine has similarly been reported to be successful in two patients (starting dose 500 mg/d, with weekly increments to 4 g/d, then weaning to a maintenance dose of 2 g/d) (Engler et al. 1995). Oral disodiumcromoglycate, danazole, colchicine, ketotifen, cimetidine, propanolol or combinations of these drugs are in contrast ineffective, and non-steroidal antiphlogistics (indomethacin, aspirin) have only a minor effect, although they can reduce the pain in already existing lesions (Schafer 1995). Elimination of specific food allergens identified by a positive delayed skin test caused remission in a group of patients managed by Davis et al. (1986). These findings could however not be reproduced in our patient group (Czarnetzki et al. 1987), although a low-pseudoallergen diet has been found by us to be effective in one patient (unpublished), and Rajka and Møre (1985) have reported a strict diet to be beneficial in two of their patients. Avoidance of provocation of the lesions remains the most important therapeutic measure. Reduction of the intensity of pressure is also helpful. Patients can be told that local pressure can be reduced by application of weights over a larger area, for example by choosing broad belts for their bags. Cushioning can also reduce pressure, for example in shoes. In case of severe symptomatology that cannot be reduced by these measures, patients may be forced to change their job.

5.4
Cold Urticaria

A. MÖLLER and B.M. HENZ

5.4.1
Definition and Classification

Cold urticaria is defined as an urticarial reaction or angioedema on exposure to the cold. Lesions can be provoked through contact with firm cold bodies, cold fluid or cold air with a chilling effect of the skin and a sometimes lowering of the central body temperature. In 96% of patients with cold urticaria, the disease is idiopathic. However, compared to other forms of physical urticaria, it occurs more often secondarily, i.e. together with infectious, neoplastic or immunologic diseases. In these cases, abnormal body proteins altered by cold temperatures most likely act as antigens. There are several other, very rare types of cold urticaria. Familial delayed cold urticaria is very rare and is transmitted by autosomal dominant inheritance. Systemic familial cold urticaria, of which about a dozen families have been described until now, manifests itself as a maculopapular rush on response to cold wind and not as urticaria so that this disease is a misnomer and should not be confused with cold urticaria.

Cold urticaria is classified on the basis of the eliciting stimuli and the type of reaction

I. Reactions to cold with positive local tests
   1. Immediate cold urticaria
   2. Delayed cold urticaria
   3. Cold-dependent dermographic urticaria
   4. Localized cold urticaria
   5. Localized reflex cold urticaria
   6. Perifollicular cold urticaria
   7. Familial delayed cold urticaria

II. Cold urticaria with only generalized responses
   1. Cold wind and air urticaria
   2. Cholinergic cold urticaria

Another classification is base on the severity of symptoms (Wanderer 1995):
Type I – localized urticaria and angioedema
Type II – systemic reactions with hypotensive symptoms
Type III – severe systemic reactions with fainting, disorientation and shock

5.4.2 Epidemiology

Among physical urticarias, the frequency of cold urticaria varies between 5.2–33.8%, with a higher incidence in cold climates. The incidence in women is twice that of men. The peak age incidence is between 20 and 30 years and the mean age of onset between 18 to 25 years (range 3 months to 74 years). The mean duration of the disease is 4.2 years, with improvement or remission in 50% of patients within 5 years (Henquet et al. 1992, Möller et al. 1996). In patients with secondary cold urticaria, the mean age of onset is higher (49 years) (Wanderer 1995).

Patients with cold urticaria come to see a physician only when the symptoms are incapacitating. For this reason, the disease is diagnosed more frequently during the cold season and in cold climates. There are, however, also reports on its occurrence in tropical regions since it is not the absolute temperature but rather changes in temperature that provoke the symptoms. Occasionally, cold urticaria is diagnosed accidentally in patients suspected to suffer from chronic urticaria.

5.4.3 Clinical Manifestations

Cutaneous Reactions

Lesions of cold urticaria are provoked by direct contact of the skin or the mucous membranes with cold objects, cold water or ice, cold air, cold wind or cold solid food and beverages. Cold temperatures developing because of evaporation, even after sweating, can also provoke symptoms. Lesions can be either limited exactly to the site of contact or generalized, and they often appear only a few minutes after cold exposure on rewarming.

The initial changes on the skin present as redness, followed by a rapidly developing whealing reaction, with surrounding erythema (Fig. 5.6) and associated mild to moderate itching. During bathing in cold water or after leaving the water, extensive diffuse erythema and edema, also with confluent lesions, can develop over large areas of the body. Often, the large edematous areas are studded with small wheals, as frequently also observed in heat urticaria (Fig. 5.7). In severe cases, the oral mucous membranes and the tongue can be involved as well. With reactions to cold air, lesions appear mostly at the time of shivering. In general, lesions develop more rapidly, the lower the eliciting temperature, and they disappear slowly within 30 minutes to one hour, maximally after 3 hours.

In about 80% of patients, residual mild purpura can be observed at sites of most intense involvement. This purpura can at times be severe and extensive,

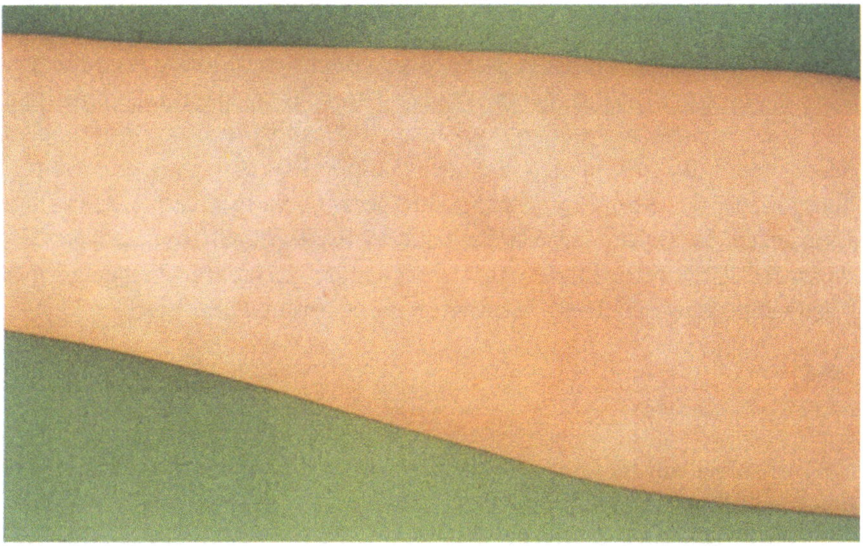

Fig. 5.6. Wheal with associated reflex erythema after testing with an ice-cube test

with subsequent ulceration. Angioedemas are observed in 73% of patients in association with whealing.

In contrast to *immediate cold urticaria* where wheals appear within a few minutes after cold exposure in the area of contact, with disappearance after 3 hours, lesions of *delayed cold urticaria* appear after a latency of 3 to maximally 24 hours after cold exposure and can persist over many hours.

In *cold induced dermographic urticaria*, small wheals appear in skin exposed to the cold only on additional mechanical irritation such as scratching or rubbing. *Localized cold urticaria* can only be elicited in certain skin areas. In *cold reflex urticaria*, small transient, but also larger wheals develop only in the vicinity of the area of contact. *Follicular cold urticaria* is a rare, recently described subtype of cold urticaria, with wheals appearing at sites of cold contact in a perifollicular distribution. In autosomal-dominant *delayed familial cold urticaria*, deep red swellings appear only after 9–18 h at sites of contact, without previous early reactions.

After local elicitation of cold urticaria, wheals and swellings can also spread over the entire skin whereas in patients who react only to cold air when sitting in cold rooms, or to cold wind, lesions are generalized. Similarly, in *cholinergic cold urticaria*, wheals and swellings extend over the entire body. Cholinergic cold urticaria develops after physical strain in the cold and is characterized by small, transient wheals.

Systemic Manifestations

In all types of cold urticaria, very sensitive patients can develop systemic reactions even on mild to moderate exposure to cold temperatures. This holds also for less sensitive patients on extensive exposure. Symptoms include headaches, chills, dizziness, tachycardia, abdominal pain, nausea, vomiting, diarrhea, peptic ulcers, muscle pain, shortness of breath and unconsciousness. Even on moderate exposure to the cold, increases in gastric acid have been measured. CNS disturbances are also possible, including dysregulation of body temperature, changed eating habits, anxiety and depression.

5.4.4
Associated Diseases

Cold urticaria can be idiopathic or the primary manifestation of numerous associated diseases (see below). In all cases, abnormal serum proteins probably play a pathogenetic role.

Diseases associated with cold urticaria

I. Immediate type reactions
  1. Urticaria
    a) Dermographic urticaria
    b) Cholinergic urticaria
    c) Heat urticaria
    d) Aquagenic urticaria
    e) Solar urticaria
  2. Food allergies
  3. Exercise-induced asthma
  4. Insect stings
  5. Nettle venoms

II. Infectious diseases
  1. Syphilis, borreliosis
  2. Measles
  3. Varicella
  4. Hepatitis
  5. Infectious mononucleosis
  6. HIV-infection

III. Diseases with abnormal serum proteins
  1. Cryoglobulinemia
    a) Primary
    b) Secondary to chronic lymphatic leukemia, myeloma, malignant lymphoma, angioimmunoblastic lymphadenopathy, Waldenström's disease

2. Cryofibrinogenemia
   associated with connective tissue diseases, hematological diseases, neoplasia
3. Cold hemolysins
   associated with late syphilis and congenital syphilis
4. C2- and C4-defects

Secondary cold urticaria is often seen in viral or bacterial infections. It remains unclear whether these associated infections play a role in the triggering and/or also the maintenance of the disease. Since 20–50% of patients with idiopathic cold urticaria respond to antibiotics (Möller et al. 1996), infections with spirochetes like syphilis or borreliosis as well as so far unrecognized bacterial infections may be involved in the pathogenesis of the disease. Significantly increased antibody titers against different viruses also suggest a pathogenetic role of viral infections in cold urticaria (Doeglas 1975). Measles, varicella, hepatitis, infectious mononucleosis and HIV-infections have been found to be associated with cold urticaria so far (Tyson and Czavny 1981; Lemanske and Bush 1982; Lin and Schwartz 1993). Non-infectious pathomechanisms may also be involved since cold urticaria has been observed after insect stings or exposure to other animal venoms, in association with food allergies, exercise-induced asthma or other types of urticaria (Hertl and Merk 1994).

Drugs like griseofulvin, oral contraceptives and penicillin, have in rare patients also been suspected as causative factors (Wanderer 1995).

The association of atopy is 40% in North America (DeLaus and Winkelmann 1973), whereas it was found to be the same as in the normal population in the Netherlands (Doeglas 1975) and India (Pasricha and Nayyar 1975). In a larger study conducted by the authors in Berlin, the frequency of atopy (46%) was clearly above that of the normal population (Möller et al. 1995).

Secondary acquired cold urticaria is often associated with primary or secondary cryoglobulinemia. Cryoglobulins can be demonstrated in 20% of patients with cold urticaria, although the incidence of cold urticaria in cryoglobulinemia is very low (Houser et al. 1970). Cold urticaria can precede the diagnosis of cryoglobulinemia or myeloma by many years, and the disease can disappear after reduction of cryoglobulin levels during chemotherapy. Cutaneous manifestations in association with cryoglobulinemia are observed only when titers rise above 500 mg/dl, and purpura is observed in these cases more frequently than in ordinary cold urticaria. Besides cold urticaria, Raynaud-phenomenon, hyperpigmentation, papillomatosis and hyperkeratosis are frequently associated symptoms. The majority of cryoglobulins are of the IgG-class, although mixed types with IgA-IgG- or IgG-IgM-cryoglobulins have also been described. A causative role for cryoglobulinemia in cold urticaria has been observed in patients with connective tissue diseases, with diseases of the hematopoetic system and with neoplasia.

5.4.5 Diagnosis

When cold urticaria is suspected by history, diagnosis should be confirmed in 2 steps:

1. provocation testing to confirm the diagnosis and
2. clinical and laboratory examinations to rule out secondary cold urticaria

Diagnosis of Cold Urticaria

I. Provocation tests:
   1. Ice cube test
   2. Cold arm bath
   3. Cold bath in a tub
   4. Cold air or cold wind test
II. Further examinations:
   1. Serologic tests for syphilis, borreliosis, Epstein-Barr-virus, HIV
   2. Serum cryoproteins
   3. Exclusion of SLE, hematologic and lymphatic diseases, tumors
   4. Omission of suspicious drugs

Provocation Testing

Several authors recommend spraying of the skin with *ethyl chloride* as a screening test in the office. More reliable and specific as well as generally more used and also very simple is the *ice cube test*. Pieces of ice suspended in cold water are placed into a plastic bag, a mug or a copper cylinder and left on the lower arm for 3–5 minutes. In milder cold urticaria, exposure may have to be extended to 10 or even 20 minutes. According to Neittanmäki (1985), reactions occur in 76% of patients after 10 and in 100% after 20 minutes. The test is positive when a wheal or angioedema develop on rewarming of the skin.

The determination of the minimum time until induction of whealing (*cold stimulation time*) can be useful for following the course of the disease and the effect of therapy. Exposure tests are e.g. started with 10 minutes and subsequent shorter times of exposure at different sites of the skin until an exposure time is reached at which no more whealing is observed. On extended cold contact exposure, one has to be careful not to induce cold injury which can mimic a positive reaction since cutaneous edema may occur as well.

A copper cylinder with a built-in thermostat to maintain the temperature allows for a more refined testing for cold urticaria. This instrument has the further advantage that only a small area of the skin is exposed and that several temperatures can be tested simultaneously.

In all these test methods, the plastic bag or the copper cylinder protects the skin from direct contact with ice and water and allows thus for the distinction of cold urticaria from aquagenic urticaria. One must however watch for water of condensation on the outer surface of the test instruments, particularly at a high relative humidity.

When the ice cube and the copper cylinder tests are negative, a cold water test should be performed. It is conducted by placing the patient's arm for up to 15 minutes in a water bath of 8–10 °C. In case this test is also negative, it can be repeated at 21 °C, since some patients react only at these higher temperature. If it is again negative, a cool bath in a tub should be done. During all these tests, the patient should be watched since massive histamine release might result, with ensueing anaphylactic shock. An advantage of the arm test is the possibility of placing a tourniquet on the exposed extremity, thus allowing for a limitation of systemic reactions. The disadvantage of all tests with water is the inability to differentiate reactions due to aquagenic urticaria.

When the ice cube as well as the cold water tests are negative, as is possible in generalized cold urticaria, a cold air or cold wind test should be done. It is conducted by having the patient sit in a cold room at 4 °C with only light clothing. Generalized urticaria develops typically when the patient starts shivering. If a cold room is not available and if the individual is particularly sensitive, provocation is also possible on exposure to a cold draft, a cold ventilator or a cold hair dryer.

The relative value of the different test procedures is difficult to ascertain from the literature since in most studies, only one of the test types was used. Since in individual patients, only one of the methods may give positive results, one should be familiar with all different test possibilities.

Further Examinations

Besides cold tests, the following laboratory examinations should be done routinely in all patients with cold urticaria: Serology for syphilis, borreliosis, HIV- and Epstein-Barr-viral infections, tests to rule out SLE, as well as determinations of cryoglobulins, cold agglutinins, cryofibrinogens and cryohemolysins. Hematologic or lymphatic diseases should be excluded by clinical and laboratory examinations. In case of suspected drug-induced cold urticaria, the particular drug should be omitted or substituted.

5.4.6 Differential Diagnosis

Other types of urticaria (see below) can usually be excluded by a careful history, with questioning regarding the appearance of the wheals, their temporal evolution and the specific elicitors. If a patient has observed for example that his urticaria develops in association with bathing, he should be asked whether the wheals develop while swimming in cold water or only after drying with a towel. In the latter case, one must consider the diagnosis of dermographic urticaria or even vibratory angioedema. Aquagenic urticaria should be ruled out on further questioning regarding the size of the wheal and the elicitation under different circumstances like a warm shower.

Pruritus or *prurigo hiemalis* (cold itch) is seen preferentially in men during the cold season. Patients typically develop itching on the extremities on rewarming after cold exposure, without visible skin changes. Cold tests are negative, but the symptoms are reproducible when the natural circumstances of their elicitation are imitated. Two rare and unusual reactions are *cold erythema* which is associated with itching but no whealing, and *cold pruritus* which shows no skin changes initially but may present as papules after rewarming. Both conditions are probably abortive types of cold urticaria.

Differential Diagnosis of Cold Urticaria

1. Other types of urticaria like
   a) Dermographic urticaria
   b) Vibratory angioedema
   c) Aquagenic urticaria
2. Abortive forms of cold urticaria like
   a) Pruritus (prurigo) hiemalis
   b) Cold erythema
   c) Cold pruritus
3. Cold panniculitis

Cold panniculitis may be mistaken for delayed cold urticaria because of its clinical appearance. The disease occurs most often in children, but also in young or older adults. Lesions appear 6–72 h after cold contact and present as painful deep swellings which resolve with a mild residual hyperpigmentation. Fat necrosis has also been observed. Cold panniculitis cannot be differentiated from delayed cold urticaria clinically, but on biopsy, it shows a lymphohistiocytic infiltrate in the deep fat, with scattered eosinophils. In cold urticaria, the upper and mid dermis are primarily involved instead.

5.4.7
Therapy

The most important aspect of treatment (see below) is a diligent education of patients or their parents regarding avoidance of potentially life-threatening situations during ingestion of ice-cream, the intake of cold beverages or a jump into cold water. Patients reacting within 3 minutes on cold testing are particularly in danger, although even patients with a negative cold water test have supposedly suffered severe systemic anaphylactic reactions during bathing.

Therapy of Cold Urticaria

1. Patient education
2. Therapy of underlying diseases (trial with antibiotics)
3. Avoidance of cold exposure
4. Symptomatic therapy with H_1-antihistamines
5. Stanozolol/danazole
6. Sulfones or dapsone
7. β_2-Sympathomimetics and aminophylline
8. Induction of cold tolerance
9. Omission of suspected drugs

Special precautionary measures must be undertaken when the patient needs surgery. The temperature of the operating room may have to be increased and intravenous infusions prewarmed to 37 °C. In addition, patients should be pretreated with H_1- and H_2-blockers.

Highly sensitive patients should always carry a kit with them, containing adrenalin and steroid tablets for self-treatment.

Since up to 50% of patients respond to a two week treatment with penicillin, this treatment should be tried in each case. After we had observed remission in a patient with penicillin allergy and increased borreliosis titers after tetracycline treatment, we have used tetracyclines in further patients and have obtained a similar response rate as with penicillin (Möller et al. 1996). In patients with secondary cold urticaria, the basic underlying disease must first be treated, and if the diagnosis is correct, cold urticaria should resolve soon thereafter.

H_1-antihistamines can be used to decrease the symptomatology in patients with cold urticaria. In clinical studies, patients have responded very differently to the diverse preparations. In the older literature, the treatment of choice was cyproheptadine, a potent H_1-blocker and serotonin antagonist with additional mild anticholinergic effects (Sigler et al. 1980). This preferential efficacy could not be supported with newer studies (Haustein and Kirchhoff 1984). Ketotifen which was similarly recommended has additional problems with weight gain (Haustein and Kirchhoff 1984). In a comparative study of the very potent H_1-blocker doxepin (30 mg/d) and hydroxyzine (40 mg/d) with cinnarizine (30 mg/d), all 3 drugs were equally effective and better than placebo (Neittanmäki et al. 1984). Moderate to good responses have also been observed with the newer non-sedating H_1-antihistamines (Villas-Martinez et al. 1992). Oral disodium cromoglycate is however not effective, probably because of insufficient absorption (Haustein and Kirchhoff 1984). The combination of H_1 and H_2-blockers is not superior to H_1-blockers alone.

In patients with severe involvement who fail to respond sufficiently to H_1-antihistamines, a trial with sulfones like dapsone may be worthwhile. Ormerod et al. (1993) also reported an improvement of familial cold urticaria after treatment with stanozolol. Short-time treatment with moderate doses of corticosteroids (20–25 mg for 1–5 days) suppresses symptoms only partially (Kobza-Black et al. 1981). Interferon α (3 × 3 million units/week) caused no improvement in one of our patients after a 6 weeks treatment (unpublished). Recently, good results have been reported with a combination of β-sympathomimetic and aminophyllin-containing drugs (Husz et al. 1994). If the patient is highly motivated and cooperative, the refractory period after cold exposure which may last for several days can be put to good use (Henquet et al. 1992). Induction of cold tolerance must be done in hospitalized patients and with concomitant antihistamine treatment. The patient is exposed several times daily to cold water, increasing each time the exposed body surfaces and the duration of exposure as well as gradually decreasing the temperature, until the patient tolerates one or two cold showers or a full bath per day. Initial temperatures should be 5 °C above the highest temperature determined by provocations during skin testing. Despite great care, anaphylactic symptoms can develop repeatedly during the phase of induction so that the patient needs to be constantly observed during the exposures. If he fails to maintain treatment on a daily or alternative day basis, cold tolerance is lost and reexposure can lead to dangerous anaphylactic reactions. The patient should be warned accordingly. In our own experience and as also reported in the literature (Wanderer 1995), no patient maintains this therapy over an extended period of time because it proves to be difficult in daily life, and it is also disagreeable.

5.5
Heat Contact Urticaria

B. Cremer and B. M. Henz

5.5.1
Definition and Causes

Heat urticaria is elicited after direct contact of the skin with warm or hot objects. Eliciting factors are all stimulants which induce a feeling of warmth on the skin.

5.5.2
General Aspects

Heat urticaria is extremely rare. Since Duke's first description (1924), slightly more than 20 cases have been reported in the literature. One must nevertheless assume that further unpublished cases must exist or that the diagnosis of heat urticaria is often missed.

Hereditary delayed heat urticaria is even more rare and was mainly reported in young adult women.

5.5.3
Clinical Manifestations

Wheals develop within 3–5 minutes, rarely only after 10 minutes, after local exposure of the skin to heat. In patients with hereditary disease and in the first patient described by Duke, wheals developed only after a delay of 60–90 minutes. Erythema and wheals are restricted to the area of contact. Wheals may be small or large and confluent (Fig. 5.7).

Skin lesions generally last for one hour, but they can persist in individual cases for 6–10 hours or even for several days. In some patients, induration rather than the typical whealing reaction is observed. Lesions are generally associated with an intense local itch and burning, although dysesthesias are observed as well. The eliciting temperature can range from 38–56 °C. Affected areas may be refractory for from 24 hours up to 3 weeks. Symptoms of heat urticaria are particularly evident during the warm season. Systemic reactions like tiredness, headache, dizziness, nausea, diarrhea and even unconsciousness are observed only on extensive involvement.

5.5.4
Associated Diseases

There is a relatively high frequency of atopy, particularly allergic rhinitis, in the patients and their families (42%). A causal relationship is however unlikely. In

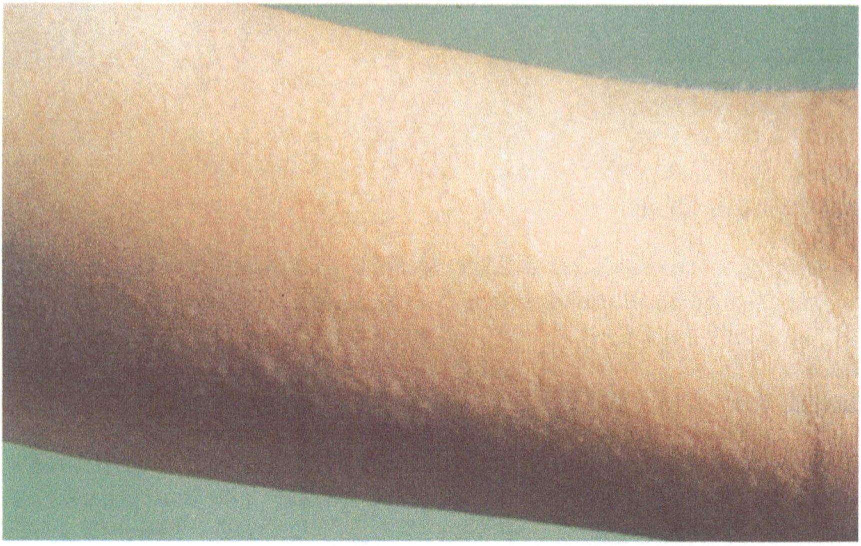

Fig. 5.7. Redness and diffuse swelling of the lower arm, with pinhead size wheals in a patient with heat urticaria after a warm arm bath

the literature, the association with urticarial dermographism, cold urticaria, solar urticaria and aspirin intolerance has been observed in one patient each (Wise et al. 1978, Tennenbaum and Lowney 1973, Willis and Epstein 1974, unpublished own patient).

5.5.5 Diagnosis

Local heat should be applied to the skin for about 3–5 minutes, possibly even 10 minutes, by submerging the arm in a warm bath (Fig. 5.7) or by applying a metal cylinder filled with warm water on the inner part of the lower arm. The eliciting temperature is usually 38–41 °C, although some patients respond only at higher temperatures (up to 56 °C). In case delayed reactions are suspected by history, test sites should be checked again after 2–4 hours. Routine laboratory examinations or immunological laboratory tests are usually negative.

5.5.6 Differential Diagnosis

Heat urticaria must be differentiated from solar urticaria and cholinergic urticaria (heat reflex urticaria) (for diagnosis, see Sections 5.6.3 or 6.5).

5.5.7 Prognosis

Heat urticaria can persist for many years. One 48 year old female patient suffered, for example, from the disease since late childhood (Michaelsson and Ros 1971). There are no reports on spontaneous remissions in the literature so that a clear statement regarding the duration of the disease can not be made. Patients are variably bothered by the disease, their life expectancy is however unchanged.

5.5.8 Therapy

Treatment with antihistamines is worthwhile since the disease is mast cell dependent in about half of the patients. In the other patients, the complement system seems to play a major pathogenetic role so that a treatment trial with antiinflammatory drugs (chloroquine, dapsone) is worthwhile.

As with cold urticaria, a hardening or desensitization after increasing exposure regarding duration, body surface and temperature can be successful (Eichelberg 1988).

5.6 Solar Urticaria

T. Rosenbach and B.M. Henz

5.6.1 General Aspects

Solar urticaria can be elicited by ultraviolet waves with wave lengths ranging between 280–760 nm. Reactions to exposure with infrared light should be excluded and classified instead with heat urticaria. Solar urticaria is very rare, although the recently described localized form seems more frequent (Reinauer et al. 1993). Women are more frequently affected, and the disease usually starts within the second to fourth decade of life. There is no increased incidence of allergic diseases and no known familial association. Causes for the development of this type of urticaria are unknown although there are indications for a possible pathogenetic involvement of serum factors which act as photoallergens after UV-irradiation (Hölzle and Hadshiew 1996). Similar skin lesions as in solar urticaria can also occur in porphyria, SLE or in association with drug reactions. An association with other diseases has been reported for cystic fibrosis, dermographic, heat, delayed pressure and cold urticaria (Hölzle and Hadshiew 1996, Laufer and Laufer 1983, Horio and

Fujigaki 1988, Kojima et al. 1986). In individual patients, the urticaria can often be attributed to specific wavelength regions (UVB, UVA, visible light).

Classification of Solar Urticaria

1. Idiopathic:
   UVB (280–320 nm)
   UVA (320–400 nm)
   Visible light (400–760 nm)

2. Secondary to:
   Porphyria (erythropoetic protoporphyria or prophyria cutanea tarda)
   SLE
   Drug reactions

5.6.2
Clinical Manifestations

Local. Diffuse erythema and wheals, often associated with reflex erythema, develop very rapidly after appropriate exposure (Fig. 5.8). The latency period lasts usually 30 seconds to 3 minutes, and delayed reactions after 20 minutes are extremely rare. Lesions are strictly limited to the exposed skin areas (Fig. 5.8), and if the dose of irradiation is low, they may merely present as diffuse erythema. Whealing and erythema are usually associated with itching, although stinging and burning are also noted. Wheals usually resolve after

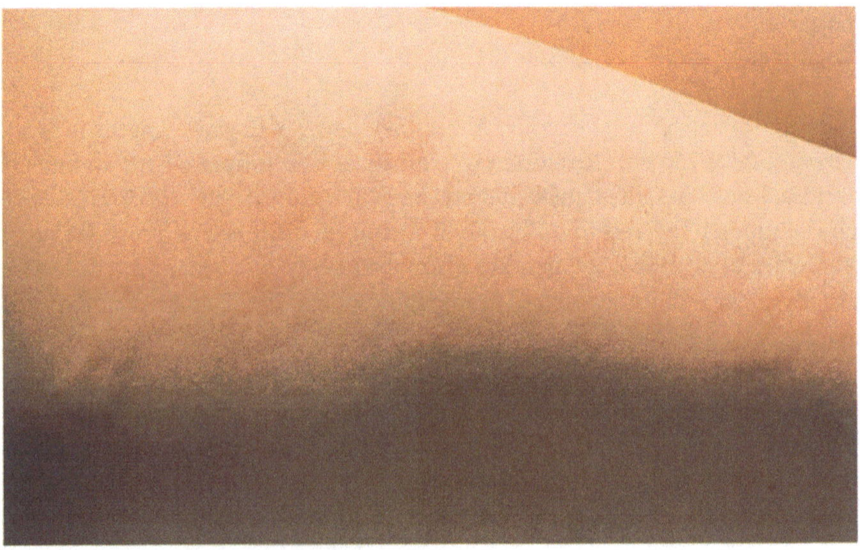

Fig. 5.8. Small irregular wheals in a patient with solar urticaria after low-dose UV-exposure

15–30 minutes and disappear entirely after 1 h, whereas erythema can persist for up to 3 hours. Areas of the body constantly exposed to light like the face and the hands are usually not involved whereas the opposite holds for polymorphous light reactions. Lesions typically appear during the first sunny days in spring when the skin has not yet been hardened against light.

Systemic Involvement. Generalized symptoms develop only when large areas of the body are involved. They include malaise, headaches and even anaphylactic shock. The mean duration of disease is 7 years among the published cases, although one patient had persistence of the disease for 48 years (Ive et al. 1965).

5.6.3 Diagnosis

Routine laboratory tests are all within normal limits. On histology, only a scanty inflammatory infiltrate is seen around the vessels, a picture that is not helpful for diagnosis.

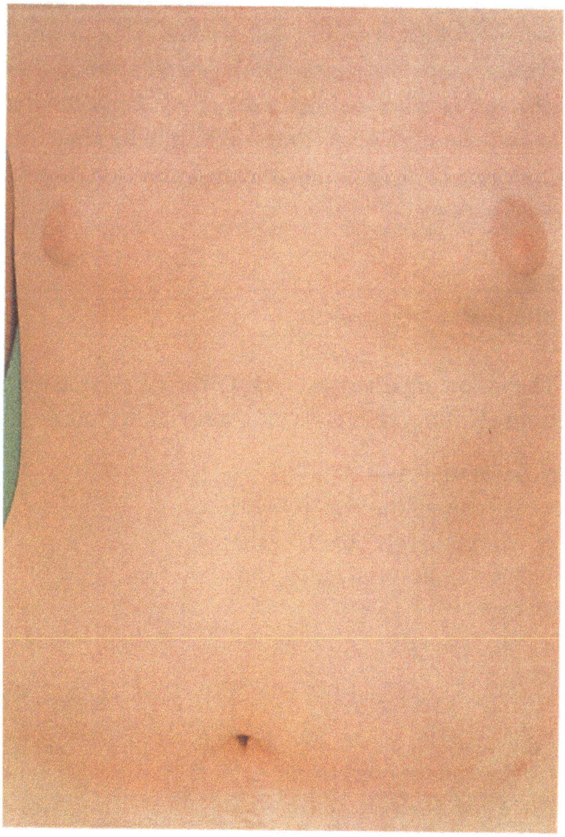

Fig. 5.9. Extensive swelling with erythema in a patient with solar urticaria. The skin lesions appeared after a sun bath. Note that the area covered by the bathing trunk was uninvolved

As with other types of urticaria, a careful history is essential. Whenever the patient has observed the rapid development of itching and whealing after exposure to light, solar urticaria should be considered. Prophyria and SLE should be excluded by laboratory tests before skin testing. If the patient has noted lesions also after exposure behind glass windows or in artificial light, the possible eliciting wavelength can already be guessed at.

Light tests are usually done on the back in test areas measuring 1 cm^2. UVB-lamps (280–320 nm), UVA-lamps (320–400 nm) or visible light (400–760 nm) are used to identify reactions to specific wavelength. With each lamp, several test sites are irradiated, using increasing doses. The occurrence of erythema and whealing is observed within 2 minutes after irradiation. If there are no reactions after 5 minutes, the intervals for observation can be increased to 5 minutes and thereafter to 15 minutes. If no reactions have occurred after 2 hours, the close observation can be terminated although readings should again be done at 24 and 48 hours in order to detect phototoxic or photoallergic reactions. A possible problem with light testing is the marked variation (within 2–3 days) of the minimal eliciting dose as well as the eliciting wave length in individual patients as well as various inhibitory and enhancing in addition to the eliciting wavelengths (Hölzle and Hadshiew 1996; Leenutaphong 1993). Furthermore, irradiated skin areas may remain refractory for several days, i.e. repeated whealing cannot be elicited at these sites during that time period. Light tests should therefore only be done on skin areas that have been protected from light for several days.

5.6.4 Differential Diagnosis

The following diseases must be differentiated from solar urticaria on the basis of the history, skin tests and laboratory examinations:

- Heat urticaria
- Polymorphous light reaction
- Photoallergic contact eczema
- Phototoxic contact eczema
- SLE
- Porphyria

Heat urticaria is easily differentiated by history and skin tests. Polymorphous light reactions are also easy to recognize because the typical papular or eczematous lesions occur preferentially on the face and neck and persist over extended periods of time (Fig. 5.10). The same holds for photoallergic and phototoxic contact eczema, for porphyria cutanea tarda, for erythropoietic

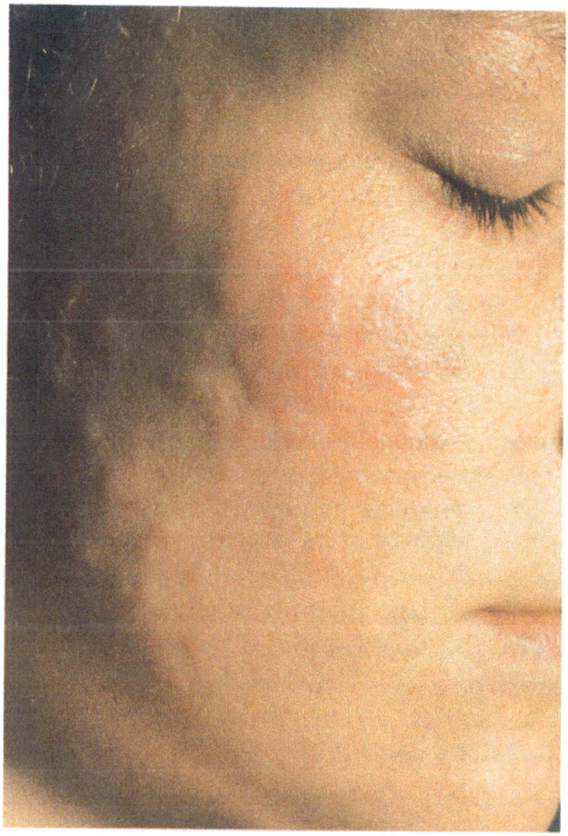

Fig. 5.10. Erythematous papules in the face of a patient with polymorphous light reaction. In contrast to the wheals of solar urticaria, these lesions persist for many days

protoporphyria and for SLE, where solar urticaria can already be differentiated because of its shorter latency and persistence of lesions.

5.6.5 Therapy

Antihistamines have been described to be generally disappointing because of lack of efficacy (Willis and Epstein 1974, Hasei and Ichihashi 1982). A trial with H_1-blockers is nevertheless worthwhile (Baart de la Faille et al 1975, Hudson-Peacock et al. 1993), particularly with the newer non-sedating antihistamines and H_2-blockers alone or in combination with other types of therapy (see below). Even a two-year-old girl with solar urticaria responding to loratadine has been described (Harris et al. 1997). Some but not all patients respond also to antimalarials (Willis and Epstein 1974, Ratanen and Sukonen 1980).

Induction of tolerance is the most important treatment modality (see below) (Ramsay 1977). For this purpose, treatment with the appropriate

UV-light is done at increasing doses at the office or in the hospital. A hardening with UV-light is generally disappointing because of fluctuating weather conditions and since results last only for a few days. Most patients with UVA sensitivity profit from UVA and even more so from PUVA-treatment (psoralens plus UVA-light), with total protection being achieved within a few weeks. For practical purposes, total body UVA irradiation, starting below the eliciting dose, with increases at hourly intervals, is most effective. When tolerance is reached, the change to PUVA-treatment can be done with care. This procedure avoids a laborious initial treatment with multiple low doses and shortens the total time of PUVA-treatment needed to reach protection (Hudson-Peacock et al. 1993).

Until this treatment is successful or if it is unsuccessful or not possible, topical sun screens should be used. Only preparations awarding a high level of protection should be chosen, paying particular attention to protection in the wavelength region eliciting the lesions.

Since serum factors apparently elicit solar urticaria in some patients, trials with plasmapheresis alone or in combination with PUVA have been done in a number of patients, with extended periods of remission in some and failure in others (Hudson-Peacock et al. 1993; Colling et al. 1996). This treatment can only be done in a hospital setting and with the necessary equipment and expertise.

Therapy of Solar Urticaria

- Induction of tolerance using irradiation therapy (UVA, PUVA)
- Topical sun screens (symptomatic)
- Antihistamines, antimalarials
- Plasmapheresis

Literature

Baart de la Faille H, Rottier PB, Baart de la Faille-Kuyper EH (1975) Solar urticaria. A case with possible increase of skin mast cells. Br J Dermatol 92:101–107

Barlow RJ, Warburton F, Watson K, Black AK, Greaves MW (1993) Diagnosis and incidence of delayed pressure urticaria in patients with chronic urticaria. J Am Acad Dermatol 29:954–958

Breathnach SM, Allen R, Milford Ward A, Greaves MW (1983) Symptomatic dermographism: Natural history, clinical features, laboratory investigations and response to therapy. Clin Exp Dermatol 8:463–476

Cap JP, Schwanitz HJ, Czarnetzki BM (1985) Die Wirkung von Ketotifen bei der Urticaria factitia und der Urticaria cholinergica im gekreuzten Doppelblindversuch. Hautarzt 36:509–511

Collins P, Ahamat R, Green C, Ferguson J (1996) Plasma exchange therapy for solar urticaria. Br J Dermatol 134:1093–1097

Czarnetzki BM (1985) Die Pathophysiologie physikalischer Urtikariaformen. Hautarzt 36 [Suppl VII]:41–42

Czarnetzki BM (1986) Urticaria. Springer, Berlin
Czarnetzki BM, Cap H-P, Forck G (1987) Late cutaneous reactions to common allergens in patients with delayed pressure urticaria. Br J Dermatol 117:695-701
Czarnetzki BM, Meentken J, Rosenbach T, Pokropp A (1984) Clinical, pharmacological and immunological aspects of delayed pressure urticaria. Br J Dermatol 111:315-323
Czarnetzki BM, Zwadlo-Klarwasser G, Bröcker E-B, Sorg C (1989) Immunohistochemical demonstration of migration inhibitor factor (MIF) in different types of urticaria. J Invest Dermatol 93:471-474,
Davis KC, Mekori YA, Köhler PF, Schocket AL (1986) Cold urticaria and virus infection: a clinical and serological study in 39 patients. Br J Dermatol 114:311-318
DeLaus FV, Winkelmann RK (1973) Cold urticaria: A clinical study - Part I. Dermatol Digest, 39-49
Doeglas HMG (1975) Reaction to aspirin and food additives in patients with chronic urticaria, including the physical urticarias. Br J Dermatol 110:382-388
Dover JS, Black AK, Ward AM, Greaves MW (1988) Delayed pressure urticaria. Clinical features, laboratory investigations, and response to therapy of 44 patients. J Am Acad Dermatol 18:1289-1298
Duke WW (1926) Physical allergy as a cause of dermatoses. Arch Derm Syph 13:176-186
Eichelberg D (1988) Desensibilisierung ("Hardening") der Wärmeurtikaria. Z Hautkr 63:385-386
Engler R, Squire E, Benson P (1995) Chronic sulfasalazine therapy in the treatment of delayed pressure urticaria and angioedema. Ann Allergy 74:155-159
Estes S, Young C (1981) Delayed pressure urticaria: An investigation of some parameters of lesion induction. J Am Acad Dermatol 5:25-31
Freeman PA, Watt GJ (1988) Localized heart urticaria. Austr J Dermatol 29:43-46
Harris A, Burge SM, George SA (1997) Solar urticaria in an infant. Br J Dermatol 136: 105-107
Hasei K, Ichihashi M (1982) Solar urticaria. Determinations of action and inhibition spectra. Arch Dermatol 118:346-350
Haustein UF, Kirchhoff B (1984) Die Behandlung der erworbenen Kälteurtikaria mit Ketotifen. Dermatol Mschr 170:536-537
Henquet CJM, Martens BPM, Van Vloten WA (1992) Cold urticaria: a clinico-therapeutic study in 30 patients; with special emphasis on cold desensitization. Eur J Dermatol 2: 75-77
Henz BM, Jeep S, Ziegert FS, Niemann J, Kunkel G (1996) Dermal and bronchial hyperreactivity in urticarial dermographism. Allergy 51:171-175
Hertl M, Merk HF (1994) Occurrence of cold urticaria in insect venom allergic individuals. Allergo J 3:379-381
Hölzle E (1995) Solar urticaria. In: Krutmann J, Elmets CA (eds.) Photoimmunology. Blackwell, Oxford, pp 199-208
Hölzle E, Hadshiew IM (1996) Mechanisms of solar urticaria. Curr Op Dermatol 3:185-189
Horio T, Fujigaki K (1988) Augmentation spectrum in solar urticaria. J Am Acad Dermatol 18:1189-1193
Houser DD, Arbesman CE, Kohi ITO, Wicher K (1970) Cold urticaria (immunologic studies). Am J Med 49:23-33
Hudson-Peacock MJ, Farr PM, Diffey BL, Goodship THJ (1993) Combined treatment of solar urticaria with plasmapheresis and PUVA. Br J Dermatol 128:440-442
Husz S, Toth-Kase I Kiss M, Dobozy A (1994) Treatment of cold urticaria. Int J Dermatol 33: 210-213
Illig L, Kunick J (1969) Klinik und Diagnostik der physikalischen Urtikaria. Hautarzt 20: 167-178

Ive H, Lloyd J, Magnus IA (1965) Action spectra in idiopathic solar urticaria. A study of 17 cases with a monochromator. Br J Dermatol 77:229–243
Jeep S, Czarnetzki BM (1994) Urtikarieller Dermographismus, Urticaria factitia, verzögerte Druckurtikaria. Allergologie 17:12–16
Kobza-Black A, Keahey TM, Eady RAJ, Greaves MW (1981) Dissociation of histamine release and clinical improvement following treatment of acquired cold urticaria by prednisone. Br J Clin Pharmac 12:327–331
Kojima M, Horiko T, Nakamura Y, Aoki T (1986) Solar urticaria. The relationship of photoallergen and action spectrum. Arch Dermatol 122:550–555
Kontou-Fili K, Maniatakou G, Demaka P, Gonianakis M, Palaiogolos G, Aroni K (1991) Therapeutic effects of cetirizine 2HCl in delayed pressure urticaria: Clinicopathologic findings. J Am Acad Dermatol 24:1090–1093
Laufer P, Laufer R (1983) Solar urticaria in cystic fibrosis. Cutis 31:665–666
Leenutaphong V (1993) Solar urticaria induced by UVA and inhibited by visible light. J Am Acad Dermatol 29:337–340
Leenutaphong V, Hölzle E, Plewig G (1990) Solar urticaria: Studies on mechanisms of tolerance. Br J Dermatol 122:601–606
Lemanske RF, Bush RK (1982) Cold urticaria in infectious mononucleosis JAMA 247:1604
Lin RY, Schwartz RA (1993) Cold urticaria and HIV infection. Br J Dermatol 129:465–467
Michaelsson G, Ros AM (1971) Familial localized heat urticaria of delayed type. Acta Derm Venereol (Stockh) 51:279–283
Möller A, Henning M, Zuberbier T, Czarnetzki BM (1996) Epidemiologie und Klinik der Kälteurtikaria. Hautarzt 47:510–514
Neittaanmäki H (1985) Cold urticaria. Clinical findings in 220 patients. J Am Acad Dermatol 13:636–643
Neittaanmäki H, Myöhänen T, Fräki JE (1984) Comparison of cinnarizine, cyproheptadine, doxepin, and hydroxyzine in treatment of idiopathic cold urticaria: Usefulness of doxepin. J Am Acad Dermatol 11:483–489
Olson NA, Kolski GB (1993) Physical urticaria. Ann Allergy 71:205–212
Ormerod AD, Smart L, Reid TMS, Milford-Ward A (1993) Familial cold urticaria. Investigation of a family and response to stanozolol. Arch Dermatol 129:343–346
Pasricha JS, Nayyar KC (1975) Idiopathic acquired cold urticaria in North India. Ann Allergy 34:363–365
Rajka G, Mørk NJ (1985) Clinical observations on the mechanism of delayed pressure urticaria. In: Champion RH, Greaves MW. Kobza Black A, Pye RJ (eds.) The urticarias, Churchill Livingstone New York, p 191–193
Ratanen T, Suhonen R (1980) Solar urticaria. A case with increased skin mast cells and good therapeutic response to an antihistamine. Acta Derm Venereol (Stockh) 60:363–365
Reinauer S, Leenutaphong V, Hölzle E (1993) Fixed solar urticaria. J Am Acad Dermatol 29: 161–165
Roelandts R (1985) Pre-PUVA UVA desensitization for solar urticaria. Photodermatol 2: 174–176
Schafer CM (1995) Physical urticaria. Im All Clin N Am 15:679–699
Sigler RW, Evans R, Horakova Z, Ottesen E, Kaplan AP (1980) The role of cyproheptadine in the treatment of cold urticaria. J Allergy Clin Immunol 65:309–312
Sussman GL, Harvey RP, Schocket AL (1982) Delayed pressure urticaria. J Allergy Clin Immunol 70:337–342
Tennenbaum JI, Lowney E (1973) Localized heat and cold urticaria: New phenomenon occurring in the same individual. J Allergy Clin Immunol 51:57–59
Tyson CJ, Cczarny D (1981) Cold-induced urticaria in infectious mononucleosis. Med J Aust 1:33–35

Villas-Martinez F, Contreras FJ, Lopez-Cazana JM, Lopez-Serrano MC, Martinez-Alzamora F (1992) A comparison of new nonsedating and classical antihistamines in the treatment of primary acquired cold urticaria (ACU). J Invest Allergol Clin Immunol 2: 258-262

Wanderer AA (1995) The spectrum of cold urticaria. Immunol Allergy Clin N Am 15: 701-723

Warin RP (1987) A simple out-patient test for delayed pressure urticaria (letter). Br J Dermatol 116:742-743

Warin RP (1989) Clinical observations on delayed pressure urticaria. Br J Dermatol 121: 225-228

Willis I, Epstein JH (1974) Solar vs heat-induced urticaria. Arch Dermatol 110:389-392

Wise RD, Malkinson FD, Luskin A, Gewurs AT, Zeitz HJ (1978) Localized heat urticaria. Arch Dermatol 114:1079-1080

Wong RC, Rairley JA, Ellis CN (1984) Dermographism: A review. J Am Acad Dermatol 11: 643-652

Zip CM, Ross JB, Greaves MW, Seriver CR, Mitchell JJ, Zoar S (1993) Familial cold urticaria. Clin Exp Dermatol 18:338-341

6 Cholinergic Urticaria

T. ZUBERBIER

6.1 Definition

The lesions of cholinergic urticaria present with typical pin-size wheals on an erythematous base, and they appear after a brief rise of the body's core temperature (Jorizzo 1987; Casale et al. 1986; Hirschmann et al. 1987).

The most frequent elicitors are:

- physical exertion
- passive overheating
- emotional stress

Rare eliciting agents are:

- hot food
- intensely seasoned food
- alcohol

Cholinergic urticaria is also called heat reflex urticaria. Since this term might however cause confusions regarding heat contact urticaria, the internationally used term cholinergic urticaria is preferable.

6.2 Epidemiology

Cholinergic urticaria occurs very frequently in young adults (16–35 years old), although clinical manifestations are generally mild (Table 6.1). In a study involving 493 persons of this age group (Zuberbier et al 1994), the prevalence was 11.2%, with a maximum of 20% in subjects aged 26–28 years. Because of the mild symptomatology, patients rarely present at private offices or outpatient clinics. This also explains the low incidence of the disease among outpatients. 80% of the persons examined by us said that they did not need any treatment.

Table 6.1. Epidemiology of cholinergic urticaria

Primarily affected age group	16-35 years
Prevalence among this age group	About 11%
Duration of disease	About 6 years

The mean duration of disease is 6 years, with a range from 2–30 years. Males and females are equally affected. There is no increased familial incidence, although the association with atopic diseases is increased.

6.3 Clinical Manifestations

The typical clinical presentation of cholinergic urticaria are pin-size wheals on an erythematous base (Fig. 6.1). The lesions develop during or up to 10 minutes after provocation and persist for 30–60 minutes, rarely even for 3 hours. Wheals develop preferentially on the arms, upper chest, upper legs, back and abdomen. Palms and soles as well as the axillae are always spared. The face is involved in only 18% of cases and can be erythematous and swollen, particularly in the periorbital region.

Individual wheals can be confluent and thus change the typical clinical appearance (Fig. 6.2). Together with wheals, an intense itching is always noted at the involved sites. Some patients also observe prodromal itching on the scalp.

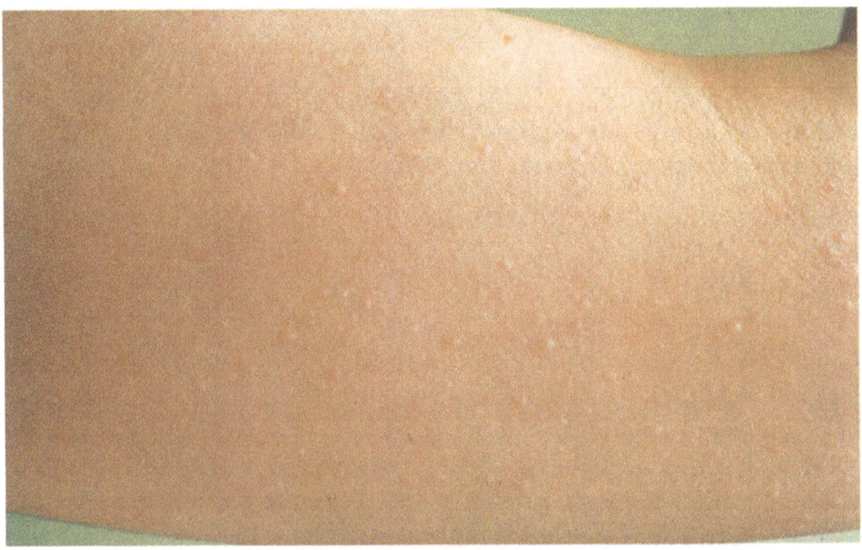

Fig. 6.1. Typical appearance of cholinergic urticaria with pin-size itching wheals on the upper arm, 5 minutes after physical exercise

Fig. 6.2. More intense cholinergic whealing with confluency of individual lesions and intense surrounding erythema

After disappearance of the wheals, there is often a refractory period lasting from 8–24 hours, in some individuals even for several days. Some of the patients experience remissions during the summer months.

Clinical Aspects of Cholinergic Urticaria

- Pin-size wheals on an erythematous base
- Symptoms appearing during or up to 10 minutes after provocation, with persistence over 30–60 minutes
- Subsequent refractory period of 8–24 hours
- Possible extracutaneous symptoms (e.g. headache)

The symptoms of cholinergic urticaria are provoked by specific elicitors which lead to a rise of the body's core temperature. They never appear during sleep. Frequent eliciting situations are running, bicycling, intensive sports like squash or tennis, dancing, hot showers, sauna, and intake of spicy food or alcoholic beverages. Fever or emotional stress e.g. during an examination can also provoke cholinergic urticaria.

There are marked interindividual variations among patients regarding the sensitivity to diverse eliciting stimuli. The same holds for the intensity of the disease, although it roughly correlates with the strength of the stimulus, the extent of sweating and the rise in the body's core temperature. Among the patient group studied by us (Zuberbier et al. 1994), 62% considered their disease as mild, 22% as moderate, and only 11% as intense and bothersome in daily life. Besides the cutaneous manifestations, severely affected patients often also suffer from systemic symptoms like dizziness, nausea and headache. Gastrointestinal symptoms, rhinorrhea or bronchospasms are less frequent, and hypertension or anaphylactic shock are very rare.

6.4 Associated Diseases

The incidence of atopy is increased (45.5% compared to 30.8% in the same age group without cholinergic urticaria; Zuberbier et al. 1994). Other types of urticaria can coexist, although they are not particular frequent.

6.5 Diagnosis

Because of the close temporal relationship between provocation and the appearance of lesions, most patients give a diagnostic description of their disease, and the diagnosis is rarely missed. The diagnosis is verified by provocation tests. Simple and reliable methods are knee bending, climbing stairs or cycling in a warm room or with warm clothing (Commons and Greaves 1978). Ideally, the body temperature should be measured before or after provocation since its rise is a prerequisite for the appearance of wheals. False negative tests can be due to a decrease of the body temperature after intense sweating due to evaporation and due to only light clothing. In case of doubt, the natural setting inducing symptoms on medical history should be imitated as closely as possible. Having the patient take a full warm tub bath (40 °C, 10–15 minutes) is a laborious but very reliable method to provoke the lesions. Differentiation from aquagenic or heat urticaria is easily done with the specific tests for these types of urticaria (wet compresses on the chest or a warm arm bath, respectively).

6.6 Differential Diagnosis

The rapidly disappearing, fleeting wheals allow for an easy distinction from lesions resembling cholinergic urticaria such as miliaria. Differentiation from other types of urticaria, particularly solar or aquagenic urticaria, is done by provocation testing. The differential diagnosis of adrenergic urticaria is however difficult. This rare type of urticaria was first described in 1985 by Shelley and Shelley. It arises during emotional stress, and the clinical picture resembles that of cholinergic urticaria although surrounding pallor rather than erythema is often observed. The lesions of adrenergic urticaria typically respond to β-blockers like propanolol.

Exercise-induced anaphylaxis (EIA) can also be difficult to differentiate (Casale et al. 1986; Orfan and Kolski 1993). Itching and sensations of heat, frequently followed by urticaria and angioedema, develop 5–30 minutes after physical exercise in this condition. Additional symptoms are laryngeal edema, shortness of breath, gastrointestinal symptoms and shock. Lesions often arise only after previous intake of food, particularly cellery or crabs. In contrast to cholinergic urticaria, the wheals are larger, and anaphylactic symptoms persist for up to 48 hours. There is furthermore a high association with atopy, with an incidence of up to 80%. The conditions can easily be distinguished by a warm tub bath, as described above, since patients with EIA fail to respond. Tests should be done with an empty stomach since angioedema can also develop after food intake, followed by a hot bath (Zuberbier et al. 1993).

Differential Diagnosis

- Other types of urticaria
  - History
  - Physical provocation test
  - Trial with propanolol to rule out adrenergic urticaria
- Exercise-induced anaphylaxis
  - History
  - Warm baths

6.7 Related Diseases

Cholinergic Pruritus. This disease is possibly a minimal variant of cholinergic urticaria. There are however no visible skin lesions.

Cholinergic Erythema. Itching and erythema arise after physical exercise, but there are no wheals.

Cholinergic Dermographism. In this special type of urticarial dermographism (see Section 5.2.4), lesions develop as pin-size wheals. They can become confluent, with possible punctate satellite wheals along lines of stroking.

6.8 Therapy

Non-sedating potent H_1-type antihistamines are the treatment of choice since they satisfactorily suppress itching and whealing (Zuberbier et al. 1995). The dose may be increased in patients with severe symptomatology. In some patients, prophylactic use of the drugs before physical exercise such as sports may be sufficient.

Some patients use their refractory period therapeutically in that they do vigorous physical exercises before going e.g. to a disco where they want to be free of symptoms.

Literature

Casale TB, Keahey TM, Kaliner M (1986) Exercise-induced anaphylactic syndromes: Insight into diagnostic and pathophysiologic features. JAMA 255:2049-2053

Commons CA, Greaves MW (1978) Tests to establish the diagnosis in cholinergic urticaria. Br J Dermatol 98:47-51

Hirschmann JV, Lawlor F, English SJC, Louback JB, Winkelmann RK, Greaves MW (1987) Cholinergic urticaria. Arch Dermatol 123:462-467

Jorrizzo JL (1987) Cholinergic urticaria. Arch Dermatol 1234:455-457

Orfan NA, Kolski GB (1993) Physical urticarias. Ann Allergy 171:205-215

Shelley WB, Shelley ED (1985) Adrenergic urticaria: a new form of stress-induced hives. Lancet II:1031-1033

Zuberbier T, Böhm M, Czarnetzki BM (1993) Food intake in combination with a rise in body temperature: a newly identified cause of angioedema. J All Clin Immunol 91:1226-1227

Zuberbier T, Althaus C, Chantraine-Hess, Czarnetzki BM (1994) Prevalence of cholinergic urticaria in young adults. J Am Acad Dermatol 31:978-981

Zuberbier T, Aberer W, Burtin B, Rihoux J-P, Czarnetzki BM (1995) Efficacy of cetirizine in cholinergic urticaria. Acta Derm Venereol (Stockh) 75:147-149

7 Contact Urticaria

J. Grabbe

7.1 Definition

Lesions of contact urticaria were the first wheals described in the literature since the School of Hypocrates already mentions urticae at sites of contact of the skin with nettles (urtica dioica or urtica urens).

Contact urticaria is defined as a rapid, but also rarely a delayed whealing reaction at sites of penetration of chemical substances through the epidermis or the mucous membranes. The disease must be differentiated from urticaria that develops on contact of the skin with physical agents.

The whealing reactions can be strictly confined to the area of contact, but they can also appear as generalized urticaria, sometimes associated with extracutaneous symptoms and anaphylactic reactions. On skin testing, the suspected substance mostly causes only localized urticaria. Accordingly, contact urticaria is classified on the basis of the severity of symptoms (Table 7.1; Krogh and Maibach 1982).

The eliciting agents are classified according to their mechanisms of action, with allergens causing IgE-mediated mast cell degranulation, histamine liberators, vasoactive peptides and amines, and substances with unknown mechanisms of action. In the first case, one speaks of allergic contact urticaria, and the remaining mechanisms are classified as non-allergic urticaria. The latter constitutes the most frequent type of contact urticaria, although

Table 7.1. Contact urticaria – clinical severity

Grade	Symptoms
1	Localized urticaria (itching, erythema, wheals)
2	Generalized urticaria
3	Associated rhinoconjunctivitis, bronchospasms, symptoms in the oropharyngeal region and the gastrointestinal tract
4	Associated anaphylactic shock

the patient often fails to consult a physician (e.g. after plant contact or insect stings).

7.2 Epidemiology

The incidence of contact urticaria is not known since in the literature, there are usually only descriptions of sporadic cases. Because of its increasing importance, latex allergy has on the other hand stimulated epidemiological investigations (see 7.9.2).

Exact epidemiological data are also difficult to obtain since some authors classify even minor symptoms like transient itching or burning of the skin as an abortive type of contact urticaria which often occurs after cutaneous application of diverse cosmetics. Some groups of workers are particularly prone to develop contact urticaria because of their frequent exposure to protein allergens in plant and animal products or to certain low molecular weight substances.

Professions with an Increased Incidence of Contact Urticaria

- Housewives
- Cooks
- Bakers
- Butchers
- Veterinarians
- Gardeners, florists
- Persons working in the medical profession, particularly surgeons
- Dentists, dental technicians
- Hair dressers
- Workers in chemical plants
- Printers, book binders
- Photographers
- Wood-workers
- Workers in the
  - Leather industry
  - Rubber industry

The list of eliciting substances grows from year to year, and contact urticaria is thus rather frequent. Allergic contact urticaria develops preferentially in persons with an atopic predisposition or atopic diseases. For example, 70% of patients with latex allergy are atopics. Non-allergic contact urticaria (see Section 7.4) is on the other hand equally frequent among atopics and non-atopics.

7.3 Clinical Manifestations

Local Symptoms and Time Course

The edematous swelling and reflex erythema of the skin after contact with eliciting agents are indistinguishable from whealing reactions in other types of urticaria. The shape of the lesions can however indicate the type of eliciting agents: a linear arrangement of the lesions is often observed after plant contact (nettles), scattered individual lesions are seen after insect stings, and tracks like from running water indicate fluids as elicitors. If penetration has occurred along hair follicles, a corresponding pattern of small wheals is observed. Since dust and steam can also act as elicitors, the distribution of the skin lesions can be similar to that of airborne contact dermatitis.

The whealing reactions in contact urticaria need not be limited to the site of skin contact, but can also induce generalized skin reactions so that the examining physician may not think of a locally acting substance and may thus miss the proper diagnosis.

Contact whealing reactions are associated with tingling, itching or burning of the skin. Particularly in non-allergic contact urticaria, the intensity of the symptoms depends on the quantity and concentration of the eliciting agent. It can range from itching only to additional erythema or fully developed urticarial reactions. Food allergens cause burning of lips and oral mucosa, sometimes even pharyngeal edema after eating. These reactions usually develop very rapidly whereas reactions on the skin may occur only after 30–60 minutes, at times even only after 4–6 hours because of the slower penetration.
The edema of the skin generally disappears within 2 hours whereas the redness may last for up to 6 hours. Persisting edema for up to 24 hours as well as reactions with an immediate and a delayed peak after 4–6 hours are possible. Formaldehyde may cause whealing reactions only several days after repeated application to the same body site. Some patients develop an eczematous reaction 48–72 hours after an initial whealing reaction at test sites. Such delayed reactions have been described with low molecular weight substances like nickel, epoxy resins and cinnamon aldehyde, but also with high molecular weight components in foods and plants.

The pathogenetic interdependence of immediate and delayed reactions is generally unclear. This is further complicated by observations that some individuals develop both types of reactions, others only one or the other.

Systemic Manifestations

After skin contact, up to 15% of patients develop extracutaneous symptoms. These include bronchospasms, rhinoconjunctivitis, swellings of the upper airways, gastrointestinal or anaphylactic symptoms. Exceptionally, these can also develop during skin testing with the respective eliciting agents. The frequency of systemic reactions is probably higher in IgE-mediated contact urticaria, particularly after penetration through the mucous membranes.

7.4 Different Types of Contact Urticaria

A classification of contact urticaria on the basis of the underlying basic mechanisms is important for a better evaluation of the reactions of individual patients, the interpretation of skin tests, the evaluation of the urticariogenic potential of individual substances and at times also for the choice of therapy. *Allergic* (or *immunologic*) *contact urticaria* depends on the presence of specific IgE, i.e. previous immunological sensitization. It shows therefore the typical signs of an allergic reaction: The symptoms appear after repeated contact - implying a preceeding phase of sensitization, even very small amounts of allergens can induce a reaction, and only selected individuals among the exposed persons are affected. *Non-allergic* (or *non-immunologic*) *contact urticaria* is on the other hand elicited by agents which cause a direct, IgE-independent release of mast cell mediators or which have vasoactive intrinsic properties. Accordingly, as in toxic contact dermatitis, a preceding sensitization is not required and the reaction can already develop on first contact. For this reason, the majority or even all exposed persons are affected. With few exceptions, the skin lesions are restricted to sites of contact, and they rarely cause systemic symptoms. The amount and the concentration of the eliciting substance as well as the localization of the area of contact determine the intensity of symptoms.

7.4.1 Allergic Contact Urticaria

The list of substances with proven or probable antigen-specific, IgE-mediated contact urticaria is long (Table 7.2). This has however few epidemiological consequences since many of the allergens have only been published in case reports. Next to latex, foods are the most frequent eliciting agents. Atopics with sensitization to pollen suffer from cross reactions to carrots, cellery and other vegetables, apples, hazelnuts, pitted fruits, herbs or spices. These can induce mucous membrane symptoms and anaphylactic reactions particularly when they are eaten in an uncooked state.

Many allergens in foods are not yet fully characterized, as holds also for many animal and plant allergens. Most allergens in food are proteins or glycoproteins whereas allergens in the medical field or in industry are mostly well defined low molecular weight substances.

Table 7.2. Common elicitors of contact urticaria on the basis of proven or probable allergic mechanisms (for further examples, see literature)

Food, plants	Drugs, cosmetics	Industrial agents
Fish, crustaceans	Estrogen-holding creams	Platinum, iridium salts
Chicken, lamb, turkey	Menthol	Nickel
Milk proteins, cheese	Monoamylamines	Acrylic monomers
Eggs	Cetylstearyl alcohol	Aliphatic polyamides
Potatoes	Penicillin G	Phthalic acid
Carrots	Gentamycin	Aminothiazole
Apples	Streptomycin	Ammonia
Lemon	Neomycin	Castor beans
Melon	Cephalosporins	Lindane
Endives	Mechlorethamine hydrochloride	Formaldehyde
Garlic	Tetanus antitoxin	Terpinyl acetate
Potatoes	Benzophenone	Phenylmercuric propionate
Tomatoes	Chlorpromazine	Enzymes:
Onions	Promethazine	– Amylase
Cucumber	Diethyltoluyl amide	– Cellulase
Leek	Aminophenazone	– Xylamase
Chives	Polyethylene glycol	
Parsley	Polysorbate 60	
Horseradish	Bacitracin	
Spices	Cod-liver oil	
Wheat flour		
Rice		
Pollen		
Algae, lichens		
Alcohol		
Perfumes		
Gelatin		
Latex		
Animal products	**Textiles**	
Hair	Nylon	
Saliva	Wool	
Dander	Silk	
Insect venoms		
Placenta		
Serum		
Seminal plasma (human)		
Mealworms		
Cockroaches		
Casein		

The already mentioned eczematous skin reactions after preceding urticarial reactions are of particular relevance for so-called protein contact dermatitis in workers of the food industry. Specific eliciting agents are foods, vegetables, spices, animal proteins, flour and enzymes (e.g. with bakers). Latex proteins in rubber gloves cannot only induce contact urticaria, but at times also eczematous reactions. Such a reaction is however not always preceded by itching, burning or urticarial skin reactions of the immediate type. During routine patch tests with suspected allergens, protein contact dermatitis is often missed whereas it is easily detected after scratch or prick tests (Jannsens et al. 1995).

7.4.2 Non-Allergic Contact Urticaria

Many of the eliciting substances in this category may induce urticarial skin reactions via several mechanisms and can in addition elicit typical allergic reactions in sensitized patients, as for example insect venoms.

Histamine Liberators. A long list of substances probably elicit direct release of histamine and other mediators from mast cells. DMSO and cobalt chloride are however the only defined substances proven to cause contact urticaria (Fig. 7.1). Other suspected agents of this group include components of nettles, caterpillars, mussles, jellyfish, chicken proteins, strawberries, mellitin in bee venom and the topical antibiotic bacitracin.

Vasoactive Substances. Plants and animals often elicit wheals after damaging the skin with their stings or nettle hairs (Fig. 7.2). The stinging apparatus contains a mixture of substances which directly affect vessels, muscles and nerves without causing mast cell release. The active substances are several types of toxins, vasoactive amines, acetylcholine, serotonin, leukotrienes, organic acids and others. Examples of plants are urticaceae, euphorbiaceae, losaceae and hydrophyllaceae. Many marine animals can also induce local or generalized contact urticaria. The best-known are the Portuguese man-of-war as well as different types of jellyfish which release toxins from their tentacles and can even induce life-threatening reactions. (Sir Arthur Cannon Doyle describes in his mystery "the lion's mane" a lethal bathing accident due to contact with the yellow jellyfish "lion's mane".) Contact urticaria can also be caused by arthropods, including certain types of caterpillars and moths, bees, wasps, hornets, mosquitoes, mites, bedbugs, fleas and ants.

Fig. 7.1. Contact urticaria 30 minutes after application of DMSO (100%). The Finn Chamber on scanpore™ on the left was used for testing

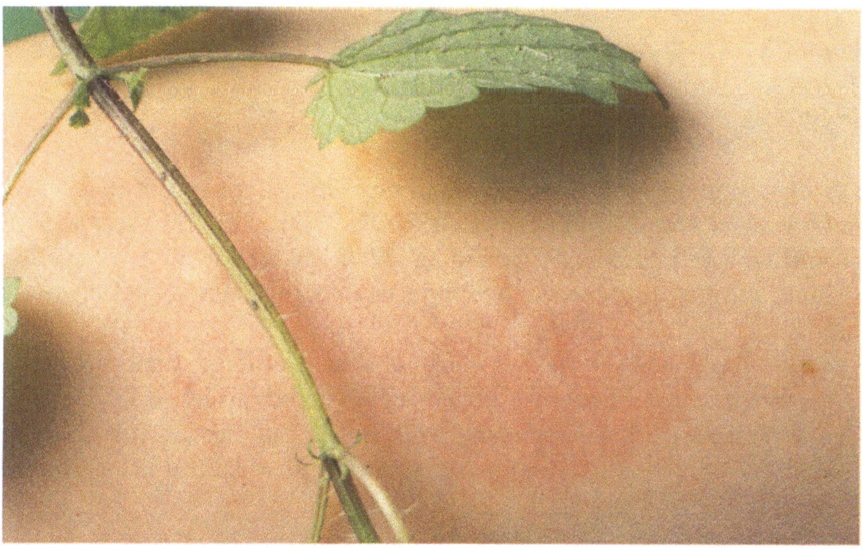

Fig. 7.2. Pinpoint wheals with surrounding erythema after contact with nettle hairs

7.4.3 Substances with Unknown Mechanisms of Action

For a number of substances, the specific pathomechanisms have so far not been clearly identified. They generally include low molecular weight substances which are primarily known as elicitors of allergic contact dermatitis. Ammonium persulfate which is used for hair bleaching is a classical example. Some exposed persons react on first contact, and passive transfer experiments are negative, indicating the presence of non-allergic contact urticaria. On the other hand, patients can develop severe systemic symptoms, and positive skin reactions are only observed in rare individuals, suggesting an allergic pathogenesis. Balsam of Peru and its constituents, cinnamic acid, cinnamon aldehyde and benzoic acid, are natural food ingredients but are also used as additives. Sodium benzoate and sorbic acid are also used as preservatives, the latter for example in some glove powders. Other agents used in daily life are polyethylene glycol (emulgating agent in several cosmetics), nickel, formaldehyde, components of plastics (polyvinylchloride or butylhydroxytoluene). Bufexamac, a topical antiphlogistic, should also be mentioned. Components of rubber like carbamate, thiuram and paraphenylendiamine probably also belong to this category. (For review, see also Lahti et al. 1985).

7.5 Diagnosis

On history and physical examination, one should remember that associated eczema may disguise typical urticarial lesions. In this case, patients should be asked specifically regarding symptoms of contact urticaria like itching, burning or redness a few minutes after contact with the suspected agent.

Determination of specific IgE is helpful when an allergic contact urticaria is suspected. It should however be remembered that this test is mostly positive in patients with general symptoms, but it can also be false-negative (see also 7.9.6). A skin test with the suspected agent is thus of paramount importance.

In order to avoid possible systemic symptoms, testing should be done in several steps, as described by Zajonz and Frosch (1994). The test substances are applied for 15–30 minutes to the skin, and readings are taken immediately after their removal as well as 30–60 minutes later. A final examination after 24–48 hours allows for the detection of possible eczematous reactions. If the patient has suffered from systemic symptoms before, tests should be done with the necessary precautions.

Stepwise Test Procedure for the Diagnosis of Contact Urticaria

(In vitro determination of specific serum IgE)

⇓

Skin testing
(rubbing test)

⇓

Open patch test

⇓

Closed patch test

⇓

Scratch or prick test
(scratch chamber test)

⇓

Exposure test on
normal skin

⇓

Exposure test on
previously involved skin

On epicutaneous testing, high molecular weight substances like food or latex proteins will at times cause positive reactions only in previously involved or possibly even inflamed skin because of better penetration. Suspected food often causes positive skin reactions only with the unprocessed substance since commercially available extracts are often unreliable. The choice of vehicle is also important: Agents suspended in alcoholic solutions or suspensions cause more rapid and fleeting reactions whereas reactions to agents in vaseline last longer. Equivocal test results should be repeated, simulating the exposure of the patient with the suspected agent in daily life, e.g. during manual food processing.

All positive test reactions to as yet unknown elicitors of contact urticaria should be confirmed on 10–20 volunteers, particularly when more invasive tests were used.

It should be remembered that false-negative tests may be due to concurrent treatment with antihistamines in allergic contact urticaria or when histamine liberators are implicated. This holds also for non-steroidal antiphlogistics in patients with non-allergic contact urticaria due for example to balsam of Peru (see also Section 7.8).

7.6 Differential Diagnosis

In contact urticaria restricted to specific skin regions, physical urticaria should be ruled out. Pressure urticaria and erysipelas must be considered when patients present with extensive and deep swellings. When eczematous reactions are present as in protein contact dermatitis, simultaneously existing type IV allergies should also be ruled out.

7.7 Associated Diseases

The association between allergic contact urticaria and atopy has already been mentioned. Preexisting eczema due to different causes, e.g. after sensitization to accelerators in rubber gloves or after irritative toxic damage, can enhance the development of IgE-mediated allergies, as is the case in latex contact urticaria.

7.8 Therapy

The treatment of contact urticaria is symptomatic, with avoidance of the eliciting agent as far as possible (see Chapter 11). In rare cases of allergic contact urticaria to seminal fluid of the partner, the involved patient can have children after artificial insemination with washed spermatozoa or successful hyposensitization. H_1-type antihistamines are only effective in contact urticaria due to allergic causes or histamine liberators. Non-allergic contact urticaria with unknown underlying mechanisms may respond to cyclooxygenase inhibitors like aspirin.

7.9 Latex Allergy

R. Brehler

7.9.1 Preparation and Use of Latex

Natural latex is usually obtained from the sap of the tree hevea brasiliensis which is primarily cultivated in Asia. The native tree sap contains 30–40% caoutchouc, 50–60% water and 5–8% non-caoutchouc constituents, including 1–2% proteins. Ammonia, at times also other chemicals, are added to the freshly won tree sap in order to prevent bacterial growth and coagulation. The contents of coautchouc are increased up to 60% by centrifugation. The proteins are partially removed with the water during this procedure.

During further processing, several accelerators, preservatives, protective agents against aging, dyes and fillers etc. are added to the latex suspension. The end product "rubber" is obtained through vulcanization, i.e. a polymerization of the caoutchouc molecules.

Latex is used in diverse products in daily and professional life (Table 7.3). The use of latex products in medicine is of particular importance because of the possible associated allergies and the increased use of latex gloves during the past years, particularly as a protective measure against AIDS.

Table 7.3. Frequently occurring latex products in daily life and in medicine

Daily life	Medicine
Pacifiers	Gloves
Suckers	Catheters
Balloons	Enema tubing
Rubber rings	Intubation equipment
Glues	Breathing bags
India rubbers	Breathing masks
Warm water pads	Blood pressure cuffs
Compression stockings	Infusion equipment
Bathing caps	Rubber stoppers
Diving spectacles	Rubber sheets
Soles on shoes	Bandaids
Car or bicycle tires	Operating room shoes
Textiles	Rubber dam
Condoms	

7.9.2
Epidemiology

The first epidemiologic study on latex allergy was published by Turjanmaa in 1987. She observed a 2.9% prevalence of sensitization against latex among nursing staff, even 5% among operating room staff. Subsequent studies provided evidence that the rate of sensitization had rapidly increased during the past few years. According to Yassin et al. (1994), up to 17% of the nursing staff in hospitals are currently sensitized to latex.

Heese et al. (1995) found also a markedly increased risk for the development of latex allergy among dental students. Only about 2% of students were sensitized during the 7th semester, but the prevalence was already 10.4% during the 10th semester.

Latex allergy is not only an increasing problem among medical and dental staff, but special groups of patients are also increasingly affected. Thus, up to 50% of patients with spina bifida have a proven sensitization to latex proteins (Kelly et al. 1993). In a recent study, we observed an 0.9% prevalence of sensitization against latex proteins in children with a history of 0–2 surgical interventions, but a prevalence of 34.1% if children had a history of 3 or more surgical procedures (Theissen et al. 1997).

Studies on the frequency of latex allergy in populations mostly investigated under suspicion of atopic diseases reported a prevalence in the range between 0.12–4.5% (Turjanmaa 1996). At present, the prevalence of latex allergy in the general population is still unknown (Table 7.4).

7.9.3
Clinical Manifestations

The clinical picture of latex allergy cannot be differentiated from contact urticaria due to other substances. On wearing latex gloves, typical wheals develop, at first on the volar aspects of the wrists and on the back of the hands. Gene-

Table 7.4. Epidemiological studies on the prevalence of latex allergies

Authors	Affected group	Rate of sensitization (%)
Turjanmaa 1987	Nurses	2.9
	Operating room staff	5.6
Lagier et al. 1992	Operating room staff	10.7
Jacobelli et al. 1993	Hospital staff	14.4
Yassin et al. 1994	Hospital staff	17.0
Hesse et al. 1995	Dental students	8.7
Kelly et al. 1993	Patients with spina bifida	48.0

ralized urticaria, rhinoconjunctivitis and asthmatic symptoms can also be observed, sometimes even anaphylactic reactions with circulatory collapse. Local erythema, itching and urticaria, particularly after frequent wearing of latex gloves, should not however be automatically assumed to be due to latex allergy. Non-immunological reactions, e.g. aquagenic urticaria due to sweating or physical urticaria due to mechanical irritation especially when wearing powdered gloves, should be differentiated. Rarely, contact urticaria can also be caused by rubber additives or the powder in gloves (accelerators, casein, sorbic acid). The often suspected allergy against components in powder is only rarely diagnosed.

Systemic reactions may be a result of inhaled latex proteins on powder particles in the air. A correlation has been found between the usage of powdered latex gloves and increased concentrations of airborne latex proteins. On the other hand, skin contact with latex may be responsible for generalized reactions in highly sensitized patients.

7.9.4 Predisposing Factors

As is evident from the epidemiologic studies, medical and dental staff are particularly at risk. The increasing rate of latex allergy is most likely due to the more frequent use of latex gloves. In addition, patients whose skin and mucous membranes are more frequently in contact with latex products and who undergo repeated operations, are particularly affected.

In the medical profession, about 70% of patients with latex allergy suffer from hand eczema. This is most likely due to an improved penetration of latex protein through the damaged skin area, with subsequent secondary sensitization. Most patients with latex allergy have a history of atopic diseases.

7.9.5 Characterization of Latex Allergens

Allergens in latex products constitute 1–2% of proteins in the natural rubber latex. Formation of new allergens during the process of rubber production seems to play no essential role. On immunoblots of patients sera, allergen-specific IgE antibodies against proteins with a molecular weight between 10 and 100 kD have been identified. Rubber elongation factor seems to be one major allergen (Czuppon et al. 1993). This is a homotetrameric molecule with a molecular weight of the monomer of about 14.6 kD. In addition, there probably exist a large number of other allergenic proteins.

7.9.6 Diagnostic Procedures

Skin Testing

For skin prick tests, the highly-ammoniated latex milk which can be obtained from producers of rubber gloves, is most suitable. Good results can also be obtained with a 60 minute extract of the rubber gloves in normal saline. One should also consider that the protein and allergen contents in gloves vary widely between different producers and batches.

In Vitro Tests

Detection of allergen specific IgE against latex in serum can be performed with kits of different manufacturors. The allergens are usually obtained from latex milk. The sensitivity of this test ranges between 60 to 80%. During the early phases of sensitization against latex, the test can still be negative.

According to more recent studies, the specificity of in vitro diagnostic tests is below 100%. Allergen-specific IgE against latex can e.g. be detected in sera of patients with a high total IgE despite a negative history, negative skin tests and negative glove provocation tests. According to Mäkinen-Kiljunen and Turjanmaa (1995), the specificity of the CAP-FEIA (Pharmacia) for allergen specific IgE against latex is 70%, with false-positive results due to cross reacting allergens. In most of these patients, specific IgE against bananas was detectable in serum.

Provocation Tests

The clinical relevance of a sensitization against latex can be verified with the glove provocation test in all but patients with potentially life-threatening reactions. The test is conducted by having the patients wear a latex glove or only glove fingers, at first for maximally 30 minutes. If no reaction occurs, retesting after moistening for 30 minutes should be done. Since occasionally, urticarial and also asthmatic delayed reactions can occur, the patient should be observed for 4–6 hours after provocation tests.

During the glove provocation tests, the variable contents of allergens in the products of different companies should be taken into consideration. If the patient is highly sensitized by history, we first use a glove with low amounts of allergens, and only if the reaction is negative, a highly allergenic glove is tested.

If the test is properly conducted, generalized reactions are only rarely observed and can be managed properly. Patients may have to be hospitalized for testing. Informed consent is necessary prior to provocation testing.

7.9.7
Cross Reactions

There are numerous reports of a simultaneous sensitizations against latex and diverse fruits (banana, avocado, chestnut, passion, fig, melon, pineapple, tomato, peach, grapes, oranges and buckwheat), with at times severe anaphylactic reactions after eating such fruits (Lavaud et al. 1992, Blanco et al. 1994, Brehler et al. 1997). In RAST-inhibition tests, cross sensitization has been observed repeatedly due to common allergenic determinants in latex and fruit proteins, although the exact nature of the responsible proteins has not been clarified as yet.

Patients with latex allergies must be made aware of such possible cross reactions to food allergens. On the other hand, the possibility of latex sensitization in patients with specific food allergies must be considered. In our own experience, neither results of skin tests with raw fruits nor the concentration of specific serum IgE against fruits correlate well with the clinical symptomatology. Proof of food allergy is only possible through oral provocation tests.

7.9.8
Therapy

It is currently not possible to treat the cause of latex allergy e.g. through hyposensitization because of the lack of suitable allergen extracts. Prophylactic avoidance of latex-containing materials is thus imperative. This is problematic in daily life since latex is present in many materials not suspected by the patients.

Avoidance of contact with latex allergens is particularly important during medical treatment and operative procedures. A change of the brand of latex gloves is generally not sufficient. Furthermore, in highly sensitized patients, life-threatening reactions can occur after use of other latex containing objects like catheters, intestinal tubings etc.

7.10
Aquagenic Urticaria

J. GRABBE

Aquagenic urticaria must be differentiated from other types of contact urticaria because of its unique pathogenesis. Most likely, water is not the causative agent but it acts instead as a vehicle. In vitro and in vivo studies of patients suggested that a water-soluble allergen of the stratum corneum of the epidermis diffuses after contact with water into the dermis, inducing the subsequent degranulation of mast cells sensitized with specific IgE (Czarnetzki et al. 1986).

This disease is often not recognized by physicians. It generally starts in young adults, with a mean age of 18 years, and it is 5 times as frequent in females. In some cases, several family members were affected. There are no data on the duration of the disease, although individual patients report a course of up to 20 years.

In affected patients, any type of contact of the skin with water independent of its source, salt contents or temperature, sometimes even the patient's sweat, will induce urticarial reactions after 5–10 minutes. The maximum of the reaction is reached after 30 minutes, with resolution of the lesions after 30–60 minutes. Exposed regions of the skin are generally refractory to repeated stimulations for several hours. The lesions resemble cholinergic urticaria in form and distribution (see Section 6.3). The severely itching, pin-sized wheals develop in the areas of contact with water, in case of total body exposure preferentially on the trunk and the neck, less so on shoulders and hips. Palms and soles are not involved. Systemic reactions or changes in laboratory parameters have so far not been reported.

For diagnostic purposes, the simplest test method is a 30–40 minute full bath at 35–36 °C. Alternatively, a compress with normal saline is placed on the

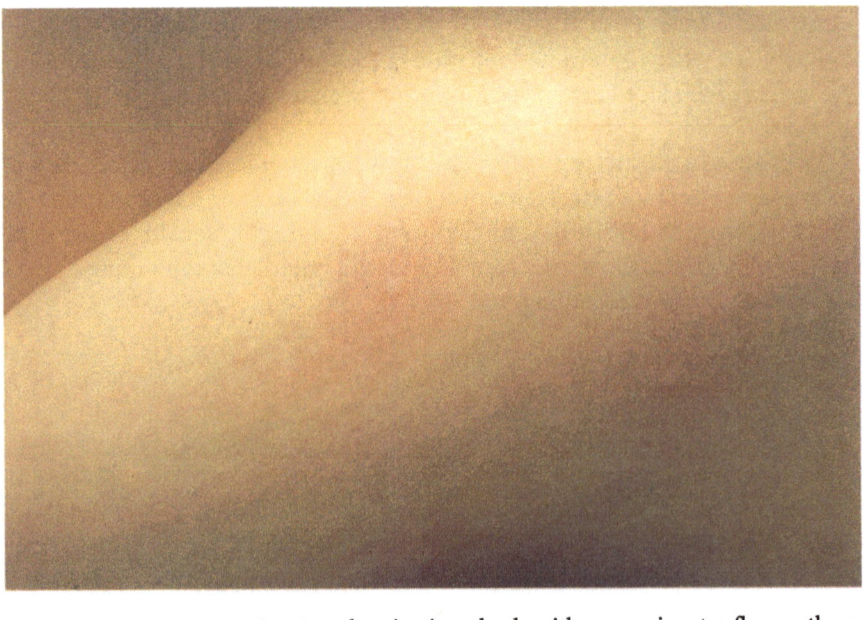

Fig. 7.3. Aquagenic urticaria. Note the pin size wheals with a prominent reflex erythema after testing on the chest

chest of the patient for 40 minutes. A thermometer should be used at the test site to ascertain the proper temperature and to allow for differentiation of cold, heat and cholinergic urticaria. A potentially associated dermographic or cholinergic urticaria should also be considered. If only itching is present, without associated skin lesions, the diagnosis of aquagenic pruritus should be made. This condition occurs more frequently than aquagenic urticaria, particularly in older patients, and it differs from aquagenic urticaria because of its therapeutic unresponsiveness. Differentiation from aquagenic pruritus is also important because of its possible association with polycythemia vera.

H_1-receptor antagonists are the treatment of choice in aquagenic urticaria. If taken prior to contact with water, they prevent or ameliorate symptoms in most patients. Patients also respond to treatment with PUVA. Some patients use the well-known refractory period after provocation of their lesion for induction of tolerance, as is also practiced for some types of physical urticaria.

Literature

Alenius H, Kalkkinen N, Lukka M, Turjanmaa K, Reunala T, Mäkinen-Kiljunen S, Palosuo T (1995) Purification and partial amino acid sequencing of a 27-kD natural rubber allergen recognized by latex-allergic children with spina bifida. Int Arch Allergy Immunol 106:258-262

Blanco C, Carillo T, Castillo R, Cuevas M (1994) Latex allergy: clinical features and cross-reactivity with fruits. Ann Allergy 73:309-314

Brehler R, Theissen U, Mohr C, Luger T (1997) "Latex-fruit syndrome": Frequency of cross-reacting IgE antibodies. Allergy 52:404-410

Czarnetzki BM, Breetholt K-H, Traupe H (1986) Evidence that water acts as a carrier for an epidermal antigen in aquagenic urticaria. J Am Acad Dermatol 15:623-627

Czuppon AB, Chen Z, Rennert S, Engelke T, Meyer HE, Heber M, Baur X (1993) The rubber elongation factor of rubber trees (Hevea brasiliensis) is the major allergen in latex. J Allergy Clin Immunol 92:690-697

DeGroot AC (1994) Patch testing. Elsevier Amsterdam, pp 301-303

DeGroot AC, Weyland JW, Nater JP (1994) The contact urticaria syndrome. In: DeGroot AC, Weyland JW, Nater JP (eds.) Unwanted effects of cosmetics and drugs used in dermatology. Elsevier Amsterdam, pp 155-168

Heese A, Peters K-P, Stahl J, Koch HU, Hornstein OP (1995) Häufigkeit und Zunahme von Typ-I-Allergien gegen Gummihandschuhe bei Zahnmedizinstudenten. Hautarzt 46: 15-21

Jacobelli AM, McCullough JA, Ownby DR (1993) The prevalence of latex allergy in high risk medical personnel. J Allergy Clin Immunol 91:216

Janssens V, Morren M, Dooms-Goossens A, Degreef H (1995) Protein contact dermatitis: myth or reality? Br J Dermatol 132:1-6

Kelly KJ, Kurup V, Zacharisen M, Resnick A, Fink JN (1993) Skin and serologic testing in the diagnosis of latex allergy. J Allergy Clin Immunol 91:1140-1145

Klaschka F (1990) Kontakturtikaria und Proteinkontaktdermatitis. In: Kühl M, Klaschka F (eds.) Berufsdermatosen, Urban & Schwarzenberg München, pp 52-60

Krogh G von, Maibach HI (1982) The contact urticaria syndrome - an updated review. J Am Acad Dermatol 5:328-342

Lagier F, Vervoloet D, Lhermet I, Poyen D, Charpin D (1992) Prevalence of latex allergy in operating room nurses. J Allergy Clin Immunol 90:319-322
Lahti L (1986) Contact urticaria to plants. Clin Dermatol 4:127-136
Lathi A, Krogh G von, Maibach HI (1985) Contact urticaria syndrome. An expanding phenomenon. In: Stone J (ed.) Dermatologic immunology and allergy, C.V. Mosby Company St. Louis, pp 379-390
Lavaud F, Cossard C, Reiter V, Bernard J, Deltour G, Holmquist I (1992) Latex allergy in patients with allergy to fruit. Lancet 339:492-493
Mäkinen-Kiljunen S, Turjanmaa K (1995) Laboratory evaluation of latex CAP-FEIA. Allergy 50 [Suppl 26]:39
Presti ME, Druce HM (1989) Hypersensitivity reactions to human seminal plasma. Ann Allergy 63:477-482
Theissen U, Theissen JL, Mertes N, Brehler R (1997) IgE-mediated hypersensitivity to latex in childhood. Allergy 52:665-669
Turjanmaa K, Alenius H, Mäkinen-Kiljunen S, Reunala T, Palosuo T (1996) Natural rubber latex allergy. Allergy 51:593-602
Turjanmaa A (1987) Incidence of immediate allergy to latex gloves in hospital personnel. Contact Dermatitis 17:270-275
Yassin MS, Lierl MB, Fischerr TJ, O'Brien K, Cross J, Steinmetz C (1994) Latex allergy in hospital employees. Ann Allergy 72:245-249
Zajonz C, Frosch PJ (1994) Ursachen von Kontakturtikaria unter besonderer Berücksichtigung von Arbeitsstoffen. Hautarzt 45:63-73

8 Urticarial Vasculitis Syndrome

W. Nürnberg and B. M. Henz

8.1 Introduction

More than twenty years ago, a group of patients was described with the clinical presentation of chronic urticaria and with necrotizing cutaneous vasculitic changes on histology (McDuffie et al. 1973, Sissons et al. 1974, Soter et al. 1974, Agnello et al. 1975 and 1976). This combination is relatively rare and encompasses a wide spectrum of clinical symptoms and laboratory changes. It is furthermore characterized by relative resistance to therapy. The syndrome is classified into idiopathic types (primary urticarial vasculitis) and secondary ones in association with severe general diseases such as systemic lupus erythematosus, hepatitis B and neoplasias. A differentiation of urticarial vasculitis from ordinary urticaria is thus of great importance, particularly regarding treatment and prognosis. On the basis of laboratory changes, the syndrome is further classified into hypocomplementemic and normocomplementemic vasculitis.

8.2 Epidemiology

Urticarial vasculitis affects primarily young and middle aged women, rarely even patients before puberty. The frequency of the disease is highly variable, depending on the strictness of its definition. In a prognostic study of patients with chronic urticaria, Monroe et al. (1981) identified typical histological changes in 9 of 45 patients (20%), among more than 100 patients with chronic urticaria in Berlin, the frequency was < 1% (unpublished), whereas Phanuphak et al. (1980) reported an prevalence of 52% (22/24 patients), using less stringent criteria. The average duration of symptoms is 3 years, although a maximum duration of 23 years has been reported (Venzor et al. 1995).

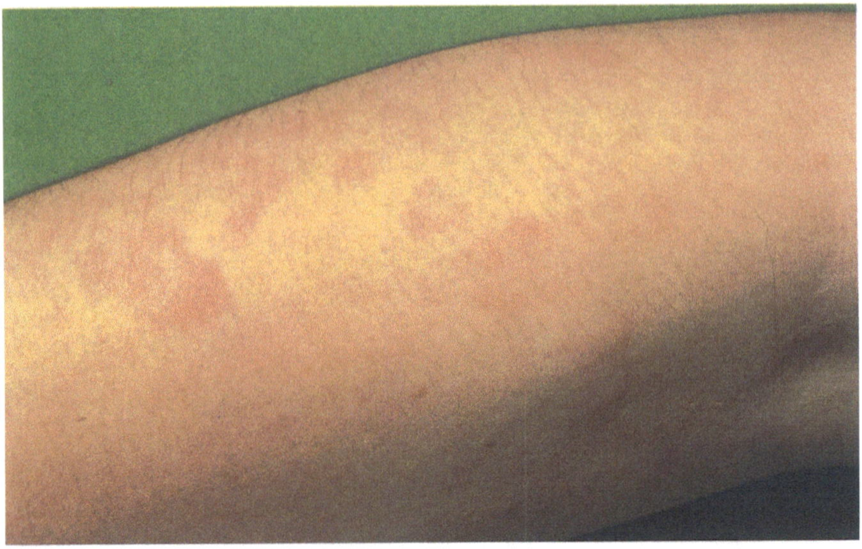

Fig. 8.1. Urticarial vasculitis in a patient with systemic lupus erythematosus

8.3 Clinical Manifestation

The primary organ of disease manifestation is the skin. Changes of the mucous membranes and extracutaneous symptoms can be associated as well (Soter et al. 1974). The skin lesions present typically as wheals (Figs. 8.1, 8.2), in association with localized itching, burning or even pain (Aboobacker and Greaves 1986). Within the lesions, fine purpuric spots may be observed, although deep hemorrhagic lesions have been described as well (Wollenberg et al. 1997). After disappearance of the lesions within 24–72 hours or even up to 1 week (Provost et al. 1980), there may be persisting postinflammatory hyperpigmentation, scaling or purpura (Callen and Kalbfleisch 1982). Besides the urticarial lesions, one can also observe bullous changes, macular erythemas, erythema multiforme-like skin changes and livedo racemosa (Table 8.1). Extracutaneous symptoms include arthralgias and arthritic changes, particularly of the smaller joints, in up to 75% of patients. Involvement of the upper airways and the pulmonary tract is of particular clinical and prognostic importance and occurs in 55–60% of patients with hypocomplementemic urticarial vasculitis. Such changes are seen in only 20–30% of patients with normocomplementemic urticarial vasculitis. In about one third of the patients, gastrointestinal symptoms and ocular involvement such as uveitis or episcleritis can be observed. Symptoms like fever, malaise, loss of weight, lymphadenopathy, Raynaud's phenomenon or recurrent headache are less

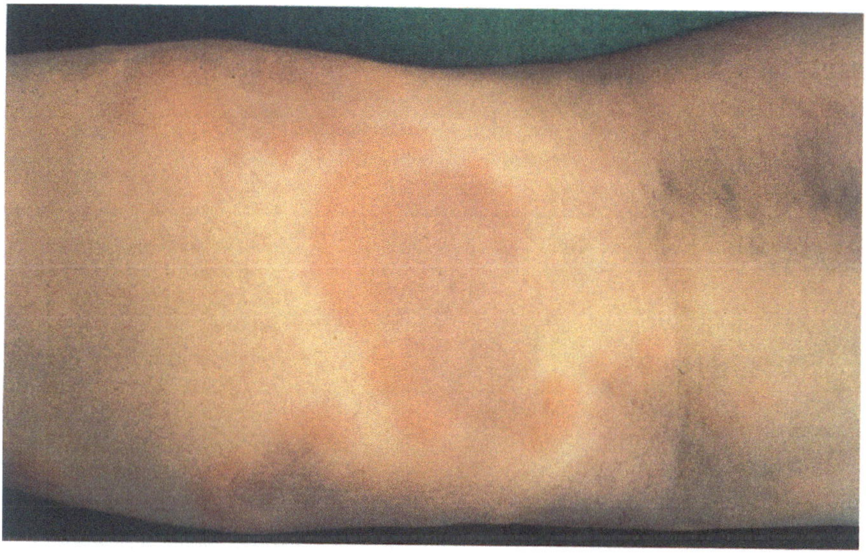

Fig. 8.2. Centrifugally progressing skin lesions in histologically confirmed urticarial vasculitis. The centrally healing area shows purpuric discolorations of the skin

characteristic since these symptoms are also observed in a number of other diseases (Falk 1984; Mehregan et al. 1992).

8.4 Diagnosis

In patients with urticarial vasculitis, the typical clinical features, histological and immunopathological changes as well as laboratory changes should all be considered before establishing the diagnosis (Small et al. 1982). On histopathology, there is a typical fibrinoid necrotizing venulitis, with edematous changes of the upper dermis, neutrophilic infiltrates in and around the vessel walls as well as leukocytoclasia and erythrocyte extravasation in the dermis (Table 8.2). Occasionally, eosinophilic infiltrates as well as an increase of mast cells are observed. On direct immunofluorescence, fine granular deposits of C1q, C4, C3, properdin, fibrinogen, IgM, IgG or IgA are observed in 30–60% of specimens along the dermoepidermal junction and within vessel walls. Deposits at the epidermal basement membrane are generally nonspecific and can also be observed in a variety of other inflammatory dermatoses (Sissons et al. 1974, Soter et al. 1977, Wolff et al. 1978, Horvath et al. 1981, Jones et al. 1983).

In urticarial vasculitis with associated systemic manifestations, there is typically an increased ESR in 50–60% of patients. These findings are an

Table 8.1. Clinical symptoms in urticarial vasculitis

Organ	Frequency (%)		Clinical manifestations
	Hypocomple-mentemic type	Normocomple-mentemic type	
Skin, mucous membranes	100	100	Raised, partly indurated, erythematous, itching or burning wheals, angio-edema, laryngeal edema, bullae, macular erythema, erythema multiforme-like lesions, livedo racemosa, purpura or petechial bleedings within the wheals, rarely necrosis
Joints	75	75	Arthralgias, arthritis of single or several joints, no residual deformities
Kidneys	60	3	Hematuria, proteinuria, decreased creatinine clearance as a manifestation of glomerulitis and glomerulonephritis
Lungs	55	25	Chronic-obstructive pulmonary disease, laryngeal edema, pleuritis
Eyes	35	10	Uveitis, episcleritis, conjunctivitis, rarely atrophy of the optic nerve
GI-tract	30	30	Retrosternal and abdominal pain, nausea, vomiting, diarrhea
Fever	10	30	<39 °C
Nervous system	12	<10	Mononeuritis, myositis, benign increase of intracraneal pressure, pseudotumor cerebri
Other organs, general involvement	<10	<10	Malaise, weight loss, lymphadenopathy, hepatosplenomegaly, Raynaud's symptoms, carditis, leukopenia, thrombocytopenia, shock

Table 8.2. Laboratory, histological and immunopathological changes in urticarial vasculitis

Histopathology	Fibrinoid necrotizing venulitis, intra- and perivascular infiltration of neutrophils, occasionally also eosinophils, leukocytoclasia, dermal erythrocyte extravasation, swelling of the endothelial lining
Immunopathology	In lesional upper dermal vessels and at the dermoepidermal junction, deposits of - IgM, IgG, IgA - C1q, C4, C3 - fibrinogen
Laboratory examinations	Increased ESR CH50, C1q, C4, C3, C5 normal or decreased, circulating immune complexes, immunoglobulins normal or decreased, occasionally positive ANA, RF, cryoglobulins, hepatitis serology, rarely: leukopenia, thrombocytopenia

important diagnostic criterion for the differentiation from ordinary urticaria and angioedema (Soter et al. 1977, Sanchez et al. 1982, Wanderer et al. 1983). ESR elevations are not observed in patients with normocomplementemic vasculitis and exclusively cutaneous manifestations. Pathological findings regarding the complement system are observed in 50% of patients. Typically, there is a consumption of the components of the classical pathway (decrease of C1, C1q, C4, C2, occasionally also C3 and C5) which is evident in a decrease of total hemolytic complement activity (CH50). As expected, the levels of C1-esterase inhibitor are normal (Ballow et al. 1975, Wanderer et al. 1983, Wisniewski et al. 1995). Immune complexes can be observed in up to 50% of patients with hypocomplementemic as well as normocomplementemic urticarial vasculitis. If this is associated with a decreased CH50, symptoms are generally more severe, particularly renal changes, with hematuria and proteinuria. Serum immunoglobulins are generally normal or decreased. Cryoglobulins, positive RF, increased IgE-levels as well as leukocytopenia and thrombocytopenia are described in only few patients. In up to 30% of patients, there is a low titer of antibodies against double-stranded DNA, in some cases also an increase of antibodies against single stranded DNA (Zeiss et al. 1980, Monroe 1981). The pathological significance of these antibodies are currently questioned.

8.5 Associated Diseases

Urticarial vasculitis is frequently associated with other diseases. This holds particularly for different types of immunological diseases like serum sickness, systemic lupus erythematosus (SLE), rheumatoid arthritis and dysproteinemias (Table 8.3) (Gammon and Wheeler 1979, Janier et al. 1989, Venzor et al. 1995). In this context, the demonstration of endothelial cell antibodies in 82% of patients with associated SLE, in 70% with hypocomplementemic urticarial vasculitis, and in only 14% of idiopathic urticarial vasculitis is of special interest (D'Cruz et al. 1995).

Differentiation of SLE from primary or idiopathic urticaria is generally easy, as long as typical clinical and pathological changes of the disease can be demonstrated. In case this is not possible, patients should be followed with regular laboratory and histological examinations (Table 8.4). SLE in association with complement defects should also be differentiated from urticarial vasculitis (McLean et al. 1980).

Cogan's syndrome, defined as vestibuloauditory dysfunction and non-syphilitic superficial keratitis, is frequently associated with urticarial vasculitis. As possible etiology, an infection with Chlamydia trachomatis is discussed (Ochnisky et al. 1991). Other infectious causes of urticarial vasculitis include viral infections with hepatitis B- or Epstein-Barr-virus, neoplastic diseases or chronic liver disease (Wands et al. 1976, Dienstag et al. 1978, Neumann et al. 1981, Lewis 1990). More rarely, urticarial vasculitis has been described in association with drug or food intake (herbs, BHT) and during pregnancy (Venzor et al. 1995, Epstein et al. 1992, Papadavid et al. 1996).

Table 8.3. Basic causes and associated diseases of urticarial vasculitis

Autoimmune diseases	Serum sickness SLE Sjörgen's syndrome Cryoglobulinemia IgA myeloma Churg-Strauss's syndrome Rheumatoid arthritis Schnitzler's syndrome
Infections	Hepatitis B Infectious mononucleosis Cocksackie B Borrelia burgdorferi
Physical urticaria	Cold and delayed pressure urticaria
Specific organs	Chronic liver diseases
Physiological changes	Pregnancy
Other	Cogan's syndrome Tumors, drug reactions, food intolerance

Table 8.4. Diagnostic criteria of chronic idiopathic urticaria, urticarial vasculitis and SLE or other collagenoses. (*EM* = erythema multiforme)

Clinical signs	Diagnosis
1. Duration of wheals for < 24 h	Chronic urticaria ↓
2. Histopathology: leukocytoclastic vasculitis 3. Purpuric or EM-like lesions 4. Clinical signs of systemic diseases 5. $\uparrow$ESR, circulating immune complexes, positive direct IF, decreased CH 50 6. Unresponsiveness to H 1-antihistamines	Urticarial vasculitis ↓
7. Serologic indications of connective tissue diseases (dsDNA-antibodies, ENA: SS-A (Ro) and SS-B (La) antibodies, positive lupus band etc.	Autoimmune connective tissue diseases

8.6 Differential Diagnosis

Physical urticaria like cold or delayed pressure urticaria can present with some clinical aspects of leukocytoclastic urticarial vasculitis, such as an increased ESR and several other cutaneous and extracutaneous manifestations of the disease (Monroe et al. 1981, Wanderer et al. 1983, Czarnetzki et al. 1994). Differentiation is easy with a cold or pressure test. Leukocytoclastic vasculitis without urticaria can also be induced by prolonged exercise (Prims et al. 1996).

In order to clinically differentiate ordinary urticaria from urticarial vasculitis, it is very helpful to simply mark the edges of individual wheals with a skin pen. In ordinary urticaria, the wheals are fleeting and change their position within hours whereas urticarial vasculitis lesions persist within the markings for more than a day.

8.7 Therapy

As already mentioned, idiopathic urticarial vasculitis is relatively unresponsive to therapy. H_1-type antihistamines, even in combination with H_2-type antihistamines, are of little use, except for a mild reduction of itching in individual cases (O'Loughlin et al. 1978, Lopez et al. 1984). Non-steroidal antiphlogistics, particularly indometacin, are useful in the treatment of associated joint symptoms (Millns et al. 1980), but they are disappointing with regard to skin manifestations. Similarly, colchicine is, in contrast to older reports, mostly not useful (Werni et al. 1986; Venzor et al. 1995). Treatment with hydroxychloroquine, sulfones or dapsone is however useful in many cases (Matthews et al. 1978, Ruzicka and Goerz 1981, Jones et al. 1983, Fortson et al. 1986, Lopez et al. 1984).

In case of poor responsiveness, the combination with non-steroidal antiphlogistics may be useful. We have furthermore observed excellent responsiveness in several cases, using a combination of dapsone with pentoxifyllin (Nürnberg et al. 1995). Oral steroids at doses up to 40 mg/day also cause improvement within a few days (Lopez et al. 1984, Callen and Kalbfleisch 1982). This is however a purely symptomatic treatment, and longtime adverse effects have to be taken into consideration (Hintner and Tappeiner 1979). Interferon α (3 × 3 mio. I. U./week), but not interferon γ, may sometimes suppress symptoms (Czarnetzki et al. 1994). Chemotherapeutic agents like azathioprin, methotrexat or cyclophosphamide as well as plasmapheresis should only be used when systemic complications are marked and when other types of therapy are of no help (McDuffie et al. 1973, Sissons et al. 1974, Hintner and Tappeiner 1979, Venzor et al. 1995).

In a recent study of 18 patients with hypocomplementemic urticarial vasculitis, simultaneous exposure to cigarette smoke was shown to be an important risk factor for the development of severe, lethal pulmonary complications (Wisnieski et al. 1995). Patients should accordingly be instructed to avoid smoking.

In secondary urticarial vasculitis, treatment of the basic disease is the most important therapeutic principle. A combination with the drugs mentioned above can be considered as well for faster symptomatic relief.

Literature

Aboobaker J, Greaves MW (1986) Urticarial vasculitis. Clin Exp Dermatol 11:436–444

Agnello V, Gabriel A, Tai M (1976) Detection of immune complexes. J Invest Dermatol 76: 339–345

Agnello W, Ruddy S, Winchester RJ, Christian CL, Kunkel HG (1975) Hereditary C2 deficiency in systemic lupus erythematosus and acquired complement abnormalities in an unusual SLE-related syndrome. Birth Defects 2:312–317

Ballow M, Ward GW Jr, Gershwin ME, Day NK (1975) C1-bypass complement activation pathway in patients with chronic urticaria and angioedema. Lancet II:248–250

Callen JP, Kalbfleisch S (1982) Urticarial vasculitis: a report of nine cases and review of the literature. Br J Dermatol 107:87–94

Czarnetzki BM, Algermissen B, Jeep, S Haas N, Nürnberg W, Müller K, Kropp J-D (1994) Interferon treatment of patients with chronic urticaria and mastocytosis. J Am Acad Dermatol 30:500–501

D'Cruz DP, Wisnieski JJ, Asherson RA, Khamashta MA, Hughes GRV (1995) Autoantibodies in systemic lupus erythematosus and urticarial vasculitis. J Rheumatol 22:1669–1673

Dienstag JL, Rhodes AR, Bhan AH, Dvorak AM, Mihm MC, Wands JR (1978) Urticaria associated with acute viral hepatitis type B. Studies of pathogenesis. Ann Int Med 89:34–40

Epstein MM, Watsky KL, Lanzi RA (1992) The role of diet in the treatment of a patient with urticaria and urticarial vasculitis. J Allergy Clin Immunol 90:414–415
Falk DK (1984) Pulmonary disease in idiopathic urticarial vasculitis. J Am Acad Dermatol 11:346–352
Fortson JS, Zone JJ, Hammond ME, Groggel GC (1986) Hypocomplemententemic urticaria vasculitis syndrome responsive to dapsone. J Am Acad Dermatol 15:1137–1142
Gammon WR, Wheeler CE Jr (1979) Urticarial vasculitis. Report of a case and review of the literature. Arch Dermatol 115:76–80
Hintner H, Tappeiner G (1979) Nekrotisierende Vaskulitis – Manifestation als Urtikaria. Hautarzt 30:484–488
Horvath A, Kramer M, Ablonczy E (1981) Clinical evaluation and pathomechanisms of urticaria-like skin eruptions in systemic lupus erythematosus. Acta Dermatovenereol (Stockh) 62:253–256
Janier M, Bonvalet D, Blanc M-F, Lemarchand F, Cavelier B, Ribrioux A, Aguenier B, Civatte J (1989) Chronic urticaria and macroglobulinemia (Schnitzler's syndrome): report of two cases. J Am Acad Dermatol 20:206–211
Jones RR, Bhogal B, Dash A, Schifferli J (1983) Urticaria and vasculitis: a continuum of histological and immunopathological changes. Br J Dermatol 108:695–703
Jones RR, Eady RAJ (1984) Endothelial cell pathology as a marker for urticarial vasculitis: a light microscopic study. Br J Dermatol 110:139–149
Lewis JE (1990) Urticarial vasculitis occurring in association with visceral malignancy. Acta Derm Venereol (Stockh) 70:345–347
Lopez LR, Davis KC, Kohler PF, Schocket AL (1984) The hypocomplementemic urticarial vasculitis syndrome. Therapeutic response to hydroxychloroquine. J Allergy Clin Immunol 73:600–603
Matthews CNA, Saihan EM, Warin RP (1978) Urticaria-like lesions associated with systemic lupus erythematosus: response to dapsone. Br J Dermatol 99:455–457
McDuffie FC, Sams WM, Maldonado JE, Andreini PH, Conn DL, Samayoa EA (1973) Hypocomplementemia with cutaneous vasculitis and arthritis. Possible immune complex syndrome. Mayo Clin Proc 48:340–348
McLean RH, Weinstein A, Chapitis J, Lowenstein M, Rothfield NF (1980) Familial partial deficiency of the third component of complement (C3) and the hypocomplementemic cutaneous vasculitis syndrome. Am J Med 68:549–558
Mehregan DR, Hall MJ, Gibson LE (1992) Urticarial vasculitis: A histopathologic and clinical review of 72 cases. J Am Acad Dermatol 26:441–448
Millns JL, Randle HW, Solley GO, Dicken CH (1980) The therapeutic response of urticarial vasculitis to indomethacin. J Am Acad Dermatol 3:349–355
Monroe EW (1981) Urticarial vasculitis: an updated review. J Am Acad Dermatol 5:88–95
Monroe EW, Schulz CI, Maize JC, Jordon RE (1981) Vasculitis in chronic urticaria: an immunopathologic study. J Invest Dermatol 76:103–107
Neumann HAM, Berretty PJM, Reinders Folmer SCC, Cormane RH (1981) Hepatitis B surface antigen deposition in the blood vessel walls of urticarial lesions in acute hepatitis B. Br J Dermatol 104:383–388
Nürnberg W, Grabbe J, Czarnetzki BM (1995) Urticarial vasculitis syndrome effectively treated with dapsone and pentoxifylline. Acta Derm Venereol (Stockh) 75:54–56
O'Loughlin S, Shroeter AL, Jordon RE (1978) Chronic urticaria-like lesions in systemic lupus erythematosus. A review of 12 cases. Arch Dermatol 114:879–883
Ochinsky S, Chosidow O, Kuentz M, Man N, Fraitag S, Pelisse JM, Revuz J (1991) Cogan's syndrome. An unusual etiology of urticarial vasculitis. Dermatologica 183:218–220
Papadavid E, Yu RC, Tay A, Chu AC (1996) Urticarial vasculitis induced by centrally acting appetite suppressants. Br J Dermatol 134:990–991

Phanuphak P, Kohler PF, Stanford RE, Schocket AL, Carr RI, Claman HN (1980) Vasculitis in chronic urticaria. J Allergy Clin Immunol 6:436-444
Prims M, Veraart JCJM, Vermeulen AHM, Hulsmans RFHJ, Neumann HAM (1996) Leucocytoclastic vasculitis induced by prolonged exercise. Br J Dermatol 134:915-918
Provost TT, Zone JJ, Synkowski O, Maddison PJ, Reichlin M (1980) Unusual cutaneous manifestations of systemic lupus erythematosus: I. urticaria-like lesions. Correlation with clinical and serological abnormalities. J Invest Dermatol 75:495-499
Ruzicka T, Goerz G (1981) Systemic lupus erythematosus and vasculitic urticaria. Effect of dapsone and complement levels. Dermatologica 162:203-205
Sanchez NP, Winkelmann RK, Schroeter AL, Dicken CH (1982) The clinical and histopathologic spectrums of urticarial vasculitis: study of forty cases. J Am Acad Dermatol 7:599-605
Sissons JGP, Williams DG, Peters DK, Boulton-Jones JM, Goldsmith HJ (1974) Skin lesions, angioedema and histocomplementemia. Lancet II:1350-1352
Small P, Barrett D, Champlin E (1982) Chronic urticaria and vasculitis. Ann Allergy 48:172-174
Soter NA (1977) Chronic urticaria as a manifestation of necrotizing vasculitis. New Engl J Med 296:1440-1442
Soter NA, Austen KF, Gigli I (1974) Urticaria and arthralgias as a manifestation of necrotizing angiitis (vasculitis). J Invest Dermatol 63:485-490
Venzor J, Baer SC, Huston DP (1995) Urticarial vasculitis. Immunol Allergy Clin N Am 15: 761-774
Wanderer AA, Nuss DD, Torney AD, Gidas PC (1983) Urticarial leukocytoclastic vasculitis with cold urticaria. Arch Dermatol 119:145-151
Wands JR, Perrotto JL, Isselbacher KJ (1976) Granulating immune complexes and complement sequence activation in infectious mononucleosis. Am J Med 60:269-272
Werni R, Schwarz Th, Gschnait F (1986) Colchicine treatment of urticarial vasculitis. Dermatologica 172:36-40
Wisnieski JJ, Baer AN, Christensen J, Cupps TR, Flagg DN, Jones JV, Katzenstein PL, McFadden ER, McMillen JJ, Pick MA (1995) Hypocomplementemic urticarial vasulitis syndrome. Medicine 74:24-41
Wolff HH, Maciejewski W, Scherer R, Braun-Falco O (1978) Immunoelectronmicroscopic examination of early lesions in histamine induced immune complex vasculitis in man. Br J Dermatol 99:13-24
Wollenberg A, Hänel S, Spannagl M, Sander C, Plewig G (1997) Urticaria haemorrhagica profunda. Br J Dermatol 136:108-111
Zeiss CR, Burch FX, Marder RJ, Furey NL, Schmid FR, Gewurz H (1980) Hypocomplementemic vasculitic urticarial syndrome: report or four new cases and definition of disease. Am J Med 68:867-875

9 Mastocytosis (Urticaria Pigmentosa)

N. Haas and B. M. Henz

9.1 Definition

The first description of this entity occurred at the end of the last century as small brown skin lesions with associated whealing after mechanical irritation. Unna (1887) first noted a local proliferation of mast cells in the dermis underlying these brown spots. Until the 1930ties, the disease was named urticaria pigmentosa. With the discovery that other organs may be involved as well, Sézary changed the name to mastocytosis.

The disease has been classified on the basis of diverse criteria (Langer and Wolff 1990, Metcalfe 1991). The classification shown below is a simplified modification on the basis of clinical involvement in different age groups and prognostic criteria.

I. Benign cutaneous mastocytosis:
   1. Solitary mastocytoma
   2. Disseminated mastocytosis
      - Juvenile type
      - Adult type

II. Benign systemic mastocytosis:
      - Juvenile type
      - Adult type

III. Malignant mastocytosis

9.2 Epidemiology

Mastocytosis is a relatively rare disease. Its frequency is about 1 per 1000–8000 patients with cutaneous diseases (Sagher and Even-Paz 1967). At the department of dermatology at the University of Münster, 100 new patients were seen by us within 5 years (unpublished). Half of these patients had developed their disease before puberty, and in more than 90% of them, the diagnosis was made at birth or within the first 6 months of life. The male/female ratio is about equal. Symptoms are minor, particularly among children (Czarnetzki and Behrend 1981). Many adults have evidence for extracutaneous involvement (Czarnetzki et al. 1988, De Villez 1995). Mastocytosis is seen in all races and in different types of mammals, particularly in dogs (Cook 1969).

9.3 Clinical Manifestations

9.3.1 Cutaneous Mastocytosis

Solitary mastocytomas occur almost exclusively during childhood. They consist of up to 5 cm in diameter, raised yellowish papules or plaques on any region of the body, with preferential localization of the wrists (Fig. 9.1). The lesions regress almost invariably within a few years, and malignant changes are extremely rare.

Disseminated cutaneous mastocytosis is the most frequent manifestation of the disease (Fig. 9.2). In children, there are typically multiple nodular lesions, rarely also larger tumors. Disseminated maculopapular lesions are the most frequent manifestation of cutaneous mastocytosis in adults. There is a tendency to develop small blisters and bullae on these lesions during the first 1–3 years of life (Fig. 9.3), but not thereafter. Other, more rare manifesta-

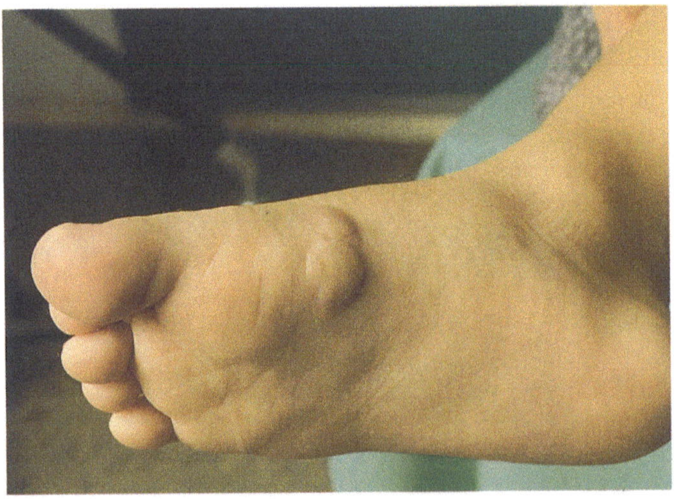

Fig. 9.1. Solitary mastocytoma at the edge of the sole of the foot. It was detected after the child refused to walk because of the painful swelling when walking. After local PUVA treatment, the child was able to walk again

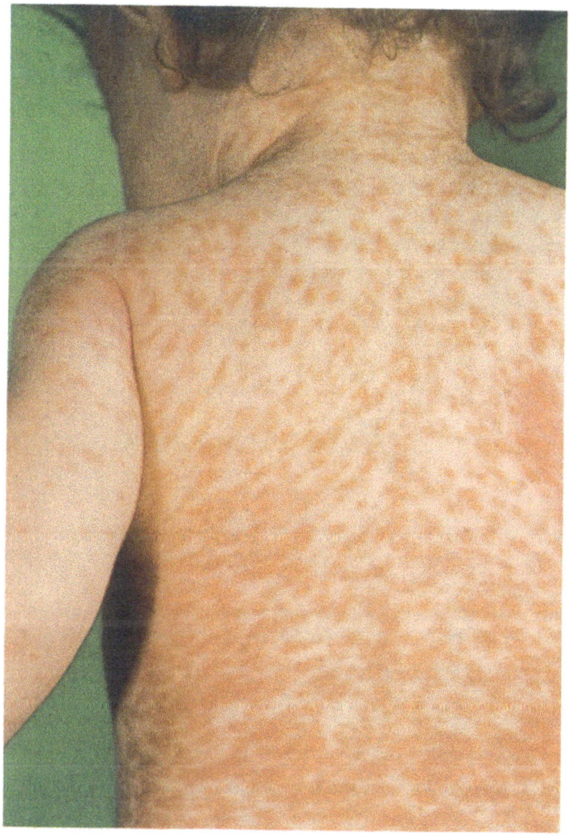

Fig. 9.2. Generalized urticaria pigmentosa in a 9 months old girl. The lesions are erythematous at sites of rubbing (left axilla, below right shoulder blade, belt region: positive Darier's sign)

tions are lichenoid, plaque-like, xanthelasma-like and erythrodermic ("leopard skin") skin involvement. In less than 1% of adult patients, focal, solitary or multiple teleangiectatic lesions, located mostly on the trunk, are the sole clinical manifestation. This condition is termed teleangiectasia macularis eruptiva perstans (Cohn and Mason 1994). Mixed forms with associated pigmented lesions can occur as well (Parks and Camisa 1988). Very rarely, persisting skin lesions are missing in mastocytosis, and the diagnosis is made on the basis of chronic urtication and increased numbers of mast cells on histology.

9.3.2 Systemic Mastocytosis

The frequency of systemic involvement is generally reported as in 4.5 - 10% in patients with cutaneous mastocytosis. If careful examinations of the bone marrow are done, it approaches 50% (Czarnetzki et al. 1988) and even 90% in

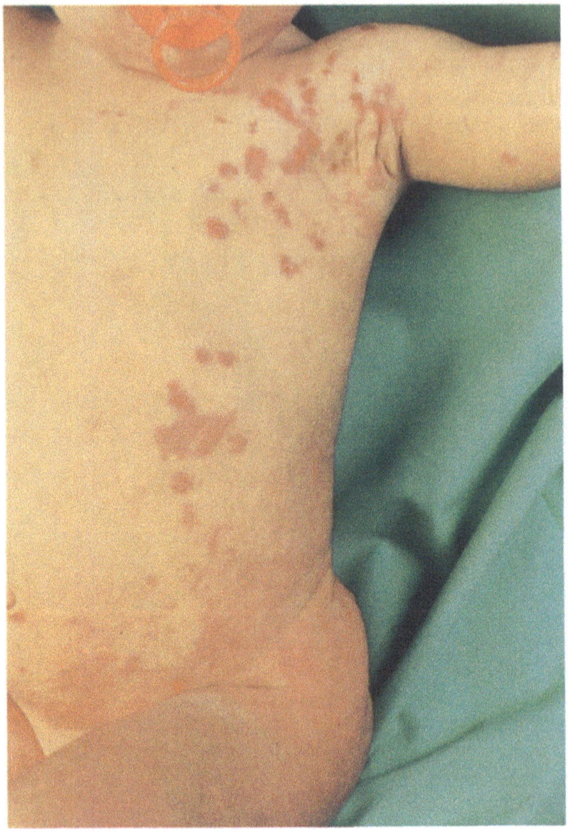

Fig. 9.3. Bullous lesions and erosions at sites of previous blisters in a 18 months old girl with mastocytosis. The skin is diffusely erythematous and thickened in the diaper area. The child also suffered from epilepsy after massive histamine release, which occurred e.g. during a warm bath

adults (DiBacco and Deleo 1982). The numbers of mast cells in the bone marrow are generally increased in these patients.

Changes of the bone marrow and the skeleton in systemic mastocytosis

- Due to increased differentiation of c-kit$^+$, CD34$^+$ mast cell precursors (Czarnetzki et al. 1995)
- Effects of mast cell mediators on bone metabolism: osteolysis/osteosclerosis

Enlargement of liver and spleen as well as radiological changes of the skeleton are observed in up to 70% of patients, while lymphadenopathy occurs only rarely. Changes in these organs do not necessarily imply mast cell proliferation. In the liver and the intestine, one frequently observes only fibrotic changes. Radiological changes can present as single osteolytic lesions, particularly on the skull of children, whereas diffuse osteolysis is more frequent in adults. Systemic mastocytosis can also occur without skin involvement.

Malignant mastocytosis is extremely rare, but is thought to occur more frequently in adults than in children (Travis et al. 1988).

9.4 Symptomatology

Local Symptoms. Most patients with mastocytosis consult a physician because of the pigmentary changes and the whealing after rubbing (Darier's sign) (Fig. 9.4). The latter is frequently also positive in clinically normal skin. Less than 20% of patients with skin involvement only complain about itching which is particularly rare and mild in children (Czarnetzki and Behrendt 1981).

Systemic Symptoms. Itching and other symptoms are more frequent in adults with systemic involvement. Flushing is relatively frequent, followed in decreasing frequency by dizziness, nausea, abdominal pain, diarrhea and peptic ulcers (Table 9.1). Tachycardia, headache, cardiovascular symptoms including shock and symptoms of the so-called mastocytosis syndrome (see below) can develop after massive histamine release and can be lethal. Malaise, fever and weight loss are signs of malignant disease. Local pain of bones and over joints, together with paresthesias, psychiatric disturbances and even convulsions, are rare and due to mast cell induced changes of the skeletal and the nervous system (Sagher and Even-Paz 1967).

Fig. 9.4. Whealing and erythema of the skin after rubbing (Darier's sign) in an adult with mastocytosis

Table 9.1. Frequency of symptoms in systemic mastocytosis

Symptom	Frequency [%]
Pruritus	41%
Flushing	36%
Nausea, vomiting, abdominal cramps	23%
Tachycardia	18%
Weakness, fatigue, malaise, fever	12%
Headache, dizziness	10%
Weight loss	10%
Peptic ulcer	4–7%
Respiratory symptomatology	Rare
Bone pain	Rare
Convulsions	Rare

Mastocytosis syndrome

- Generalized itching
- Pulsating headaches
- Bronchospasms
- Vagovasal syncopy
- Inability to concentrate
- Depressive moods

9.5 Histology

In adults with beginning mastocytosis, there is most frequently an increase of spindel shaped mast cells, with long cytoplasmatic processes in a perivascular location, diffusely scattered within the upper dermis. Five to seven mast cells per microscopic field (400 × magnification) are thought to be diagnostic (Fig. 9.5) (Lennert 1962). In adult-type mastocytosis, it is often quite difficult to decide whether the numbers of mast cells in the tissue are really increased. In case of doubt, several biopsies should be made at different locations. Recent immunohistological examinations of lesions of urticaria pigmentosa have shown that mast cells are less mature but otherwise normal, compared to mastocytomas and mast cells in normal skin (Haas et al. 1994, Hamann et al. 1995a). An increased lesional expression of the well known mast cell growth factor SCF (Longley et al. 1993) could so far not be confirmed by us (Hamann et al. 1995b). In contrast to childhood mastocytomas, adult urticaria pigmentosa lesions have a mutation in the c-kit (SCF receptor) of their lesional mast cells (Büttner et al. 1997). This mutation has previously been identified in a mast cell leukemia (Furitsu et al. 1993), in the peripheral blood mononuclear cells of patients with mastocytosis and associated hematologic disorders

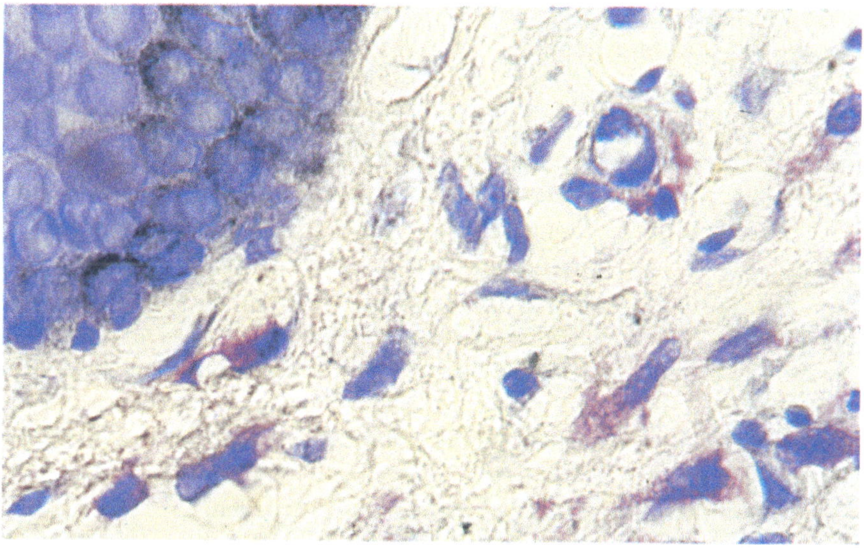

Fig. 9.5. Histologic section of epidermis and upper dermis in an adult patient with mastocytosis. Note the violet discoloration of intracellular and released mast cell granules due to their metachromatic staining characteristics (toluidine blue × 400)

(Nagata et al. 1995), and in cutaneous and spleen mast cells of adult mastocytosis (Longley et al. 1996). Thus, the presence of the mutation alone does not determine the malignant or benign behavior of the cells.

In the bone marrow, there is frequently a focal or a diffuse increase in the number of mast cells (Czarnetzki et al. 1988). Bone marrow aspirations often yield false-negative results due to the focal nature of the mast cell increase, because of sclerosing alterations and due to the adherence of mast cells to the connective tissue septae and the endostium (Webb et al. 1982). Other possible changes in the bone marrow are a myeloid hyperplasia with a shift to the left, a decreased erythropoiesis and a moderate to pronounced eosinophilia. In children, involvement of the bone marrow can also occur in up to 50% (Rodermund et al. 1978).

For the demonstration of mast cells, specific stains like toluidine blue, methylene blue or Giemsa are necessary (Lennert 1962, Haas et al. 1994). Possible signs for a malignant transformation are an increased ratio of nucleus to cytoplasm, fewer cytoplasmic granules, an increase of atypical mitoses and an increased cellular and nuclear polymorphism, with giant cells. Different authors disagree however on the significance of these findings.

9.6 Laboratory Findings

Histamine levels in the skin, the serum and the urine of patients with systemic mastocytosis are variably increased. Histamine metabolites in the urine correlate better with the number of mast cells in the tissue than histamine itself (Granerus et al. 1983, Kors et al. 1996). Other mast cell products like prostaglandin D_2, leukotrienes and glykosaminoglycans can be increased in the skin, the serum or the urine (Czarnetzki 1986). An increase of alkaline phosphatase, calcium and phosphorus as well as decreased cholesterol and serum prothrombin levels can be secondary to hepatic and skeletal involvement (Table 9.2).

Changes of formed elements in the blood can be due to fibrosis of the bone marrow and are exclusively observed in systemic mastocytosis. Signs of an early leukemia should be watched for (see below). Circulating tissue mast cells have supposedly been observed in 16% of patients with systemic mastocytosis, an eosinophilia however only in 12% (Sagher and Even-Paz 1967).

Hematological Diseases in Systemic Mastocytosis

- Leukocytosis, leukopenia
- Anemia (due to decreased erythropoiesis)
- Myeloproliferative diseases
- Mast cell leukemia

9.7 Diagnosis

Most types of cutaneous mastocytosis can be recognized because of the typical clinical appearance. Table 9.3 lists the sequence of diagnostic steps to be

Table 9.2. Laboratory findings in systemic mastocytosis ((+) = increase; (–) = decrease; Ca = serum calcium; P = serum phosphorus)

Blood	Urine
Histamine (+)	Histamine and metabolites (+)
Tryptase (+)	PGD2 (+)
Alkaline phosphatase, Ca, P (+)	Hyaluronic acid (+)
Cholesterol (–)	Chondroitin sulfates (+)
Prothrombin time (–)	
Thromboxane B2 (+)	
6 Keto-PGF_2 (–)	

Table 9.3. Diagnostic measures in mastocytosis (+/– = not obligatory, dependent on indication; Ca = serum calcium; P= serum phosphorus)

	Children	Adults
1. Patient history, clinical examination	+	+
2. Darier's sign (positive in 90%)	+	+
3. CBC & diff., liver enzymes, Ca, P	+	+
4. Skin biopsy	+/–	+
5. Bone marrow puncture and biopsy	–	+
6. X-rays of bone and gastrointestinal tract	–	+/–

undertaken in children and adults. In 90% of patients, the diagnosis can be confirmed by the development of erythema and whealing after rubbing (Darier's test). About 50% of patients also develop dermographic whealing in normal skin (Fig. 9.6).

In order to rule out systemic involvement, patients or parents should be asked about gastrointestinal symptoms or flush. Liver, spleen and peripheral lymph nodes should be palpated on physical examination. All patients should have a comprehensive blood test, including alkaline phophatase, liver and serum phosphate.

In very small children, a skin biopsy need not be made when the clinical presentation is typical because of the mostly benign nature of the disease. The biopsy is on the other hand helpful to confirm the diagnosis and to exclude malignant transformation. In adults, a bone marrow biopsy should

Fig. 9.6. Urticarial dermographism in an adult with mastocytosis. Note the irregular border of the linear wheal which is due to more marked whealing at sites of increased mast cell numbers

always be made. Other examinations like X-rays of the skeleton, sonographic examination of the liver and analysis of the urine for histamine metabolites can be done, dependent on the symptomatology.

9.8 Prognosis

With a few exceptions, mastocytosis is due to a benign proliferation of mast cells (e.g. dogs with mastocytosis are known to have a normal or even a prolonged life expectancy) (Cook 1969). In juvenile mastocytosis, the stimulus for mast cell proliferation is apparently lost in the majority of cases, and the lesions mostly regress by puberty. In contrast, spontaneous remission is observed only rarely with the onset of the disease after puberty, and it also seems less likely in children whose disease starts later after birth. Spontaneous regression is however also observed despite systemic involvement (Robinson et al. 1962, Kors et al. 1996).

In adults with systemic but no cutaneous involvement, up to one third were formerly thought to develop malignant mastocytosis or another type of malignant leukemia (Lennert and Parwaresch 1979). According to newer data and own observations, such cases are extremely rare in patients with cutaneous involvement (Metcalfe 1991). Cardiovascular collapse after massive mast cell degranulation or due to bleeding or perforating peptic ulcers can, however, be

Table 9.4. Potentially life-threatening situations for mastocytosis patients due to unspecific mast cell degranulation

Nonspecific mast cell degranulators	Beware of
Heat, cold	Marked changes in temperature
Mechanical stimuli	Massage
Alcohol	
Insect and snake venoms	Bee or wasp hyposensitisation (can however be successful when done with care)
Bacterial toxins or polypeptides in food	Fish, crabs, lobster
Drugs	Curare (anesthesia) Radio contrast reagents Dextrane (fluid expanders) Morphine Codeine (frequently in cough medicine) Chymotrypsin (in enzyme preparations) Polymyxin B Parathormon (functional diagnosis) Somatostatin (for hemostasis)

life-threatening. These complications have been observed in 4–7% of patients with systemic mastocytosis.

Parents and/or patients must therefore be thoroughly informed about the nature of the disease and regarding substances which can cause a sudden and massive release of mast cell mediators (Table 9.4). Physicians should consider the mast cell degranulating activity of certain drugs. Anaphylactic reactions during general anesthesia as well as exposure to radio contrast media, opiates, volume expanders or peptide hormones are particularly dangerous for mastocytosis patients. If these drugs cannot be avoided, the patients should be treated prophylactically with H1-type antihistamines and corticosteroids. Particularly endangered patients should carry adrenaline inhalers and/or a first aid kit containing antihistamines, corticosteroids and adrenalin spray. Although insect stings can be life-threatening, recent experiences have shown that hyposensitisation of specifically sensitized patients with mastocytosis can be achieved when done with great care.

9.9 Therapy

Since no causative treatment of mastocytosis is as yet available, treatment is otherwise symptomatic, dependent on the types of symptoms and their severity.

For itching and other symptoms responding to H1-type antihistamines, new non-sedating antihistamines like cetirizine (10 mg/d) cause satisfying relief. Alternately, an antihistamine with more marked sedation like hydroxyzine (25 mg/d) can be recommended for the evening. Flushing is supposedly responsive to cycloxygenase inhibitors like aspirin (500–1500 mg/d) (Roberts et al. 1980).

Gastrointestinal symptoms like increased gastric acidity can be treated with an H2-blocker (Johnson et al. 1980). The effective dosis of the H2-blocker cimetidin is 200–800 mg/d. Undesirable effects like brady- and tachycardia should be watched for. Diarrhea and abdominal cramps respond well to oral disodium cromoglycate (Soter et al 1979, Czarnetzki and Behrendt 1981). Because of its low gastrointestinal absorption (1–2%), oral disodium cromoglycate is primarily effective regarding gastrointestinal symptoms, although pruritus decreases also after a delay of two weeks (Czarnetzki and Behrendt 1981). The doses in children is 400 mg/d, in adults 800 mg/d. Minor adverse effects like constipation should be watched for. Long-term treatment is costly since the drug is rather expensive.

Therapeutic Possibilities for Symptomatic Treatment of Mastocytosis

H_1-type antihistamines
H_2-type antihistamines
Aspirin
Disodium cromoglycate
PUVA, also local PUVA
Topical corticosteroids under occlusion
Interferon α
UVA1

Circumscribed, symptomatic mastocytomas, e.g. at the sole of the foot, but also diffuse types of cutaneous mastocytosis, respond in part to PUVA (Christophers et al. 1978, unpublished own observations). Pruritus and whealing decrease, and the lesions gradually disappear after several weeks of treatment. Symptoms and lesions of generalized urticaria pigmentosa recur however within 6 months to one year (Czarnetzki et al. 1985, Kolde et al. 1984). Under local occlusion with potent corticosteroids, e.g. clobetasol, mastocytomas can be made to disappear entirely (Taylor et al. 1993), but they recur within a year. Treatment with interferon causes improvement of symptoms and partly also lesions in benign mastocytosis (Czarnetzki et al. 1994, Kolde et al. 1995, Lippert and Henz 1996). Impressive individual responses have furthermore been reported in a patient with more aggressive disease (Kluin-Nelemans et al. 1993) although this could not be confirmed by others (Worobec et al. 1996). Recently, treatment with UVA1 has also been reported to be highly beneficial (Stege et al. 1995).

Literature

Büttner C, Heide I, Sepp N, Henz BM, Grabbe J (1997) Identification of a c-kit mutation in adult - but not in childhood-onset mastocytosis. Arch Derm Res 289 (Suppl.): A39
Christophers E, Hönigsmann H, Wolff K, Langner A (1978) PUVA-treatment of urticaria pigmentosa. Brit J Dermatol 98:701-702
Cohn MS, Mason MJ (1994) Teleangiectasia macularis eruptiva perstans. J Am Osteopath Assoc 94:246-248
Cook JE (1969) Canine mast cell diseases. In: Lingemann CH, Garner FM (eds.) Comparative morphology of hematopoietic neoplasms. Natl Cancer Inst Monogr 3, pp 267-283
Czarnetzki BM (1983) A double-blind cross-over study of the effect of ketotifen in urticaria pigmentosa. Dermatologica 166:44-47
Czarnetzki BM (1986) Urticaria. Springer, Berlin Heidelberg New York Tokyo
Czarnetzki BM, Algermissen B, Jeep S, Haas N, Nürnberg W, Müller K, Kropp J-D (1994) Interferon treatment of patients with chronic urticaria and mastocytosis. J Am Acad Dermatol 30:500-501
Czarnetzki BM, Behrendt H (1981) Urticaria pigmentosa: Clinical picture and response to oral disodiumcromoglycate. Br J Dermatol 105:563-568

Czarnetzki BM, Kolde G, Schoemann A, Urbanitz S, Urbanitz D (1988) Bone marrow findings in adult patients with urticaria pigmentosa. J Am Acad Dermatol 18:45-51
Czarnetzki BM, Rosenbach T, Kolde G, Frosch PJ (1985) Phototherapy of urticaria pigmentosa: clinical response and changes of cutaneous reactivity, histamine and chemotactic leukotrienes. Arch Derm Res 255:105-113
Czarnetzki BM, Grabbe J, Kolde G, Krüger-Krasagakes S, Zuberbier T (1995) Mast cells in the cytokine network - the what, where from and what for. Exp. Dermatol 4:221-226
De Villez RL (1995) Urticaria pigmentosa. Im All Clin N Am 15:775-784
DiBacco RS, Deleo VA (1982) Mastocytosis and the mast cell. J Am Acad Dermatol 7: 709-722
Furitsu T, Tsujima T, Tono T, Kitayama H, Koshimizu U, Sugahara H, Butterfield JH, Ashman LK, Kanayama Y, Matsuzawa Y, Kitamura Y, KanakuraY (1993) Identification of mutations in the coding sequence of the proto-oncogene c-kit in a human mast cell leukemia cell line causing ligand-independent activation of c-kit product. J Clin Invest 99:1736-1744
Granerus G, Olafsson JH, Roupe G (1983) Studies on histamine metabolism in mastocytosis. J Invest Dermatol 80:410-416
Haas N, Hamann K, Grabbe J, Algermissen B, Czarnetzki BM (1994) Phenotypic evaluation of skin lesions in urticaria pigmentosa and mastocytosis. Arch Dermatol Res 286: 380-385
Hamann K, Haas N, Grabbe J, Welker P, Czarnetzki BM (1995a) Two novel mast cell phenotypic markers, monoclonal antibodies Ki-MC1 and Ki-M1P, identify distinct mast cell subtypes. Br J Dermatol 133:547-552
Hamann K, Haas N, Grabbe J, Czarnetzki BM (1995b) Expression of stem cell factor in cutaneous mastocytosis. Br J Dermatol 133:203-208
Johnson GJ, Silvis SE, Roitman B, Blumenthal M, Gilbert HS (1980) Long-term treatment of systemic mastocytosis with histamine H_2 receptor antagonists. Am J Gastroenterol 74: 485-489
Kluin-Nelemans HC, Jansen JH, Breukelman H, Wolthers BG, Kluin PM, Kroon HM, Willemze R (1993) Response of interferon α-2β in a patient with systemic mastocytosis. N Engl Med 326:619-623
Kolde G, Frosch PJ, Czarnetzki BM (1984) Response of cutaneous mast cells to PUVA in patients with urticaria pigmentosa. Histomorphometric, ultrastructural and biochemical investigations. J Invest Dermatol 83:175-178
Kolde G, Sunderkötter C, Luger TA (1995) Treatment of urticaria pigmentosa using interferon alpha. Br J Dermatol 133:91-94
Kors JW, Van Doormaal JJ, Breukelman H, Van Voorst Vader PC, De Monchy JGR (1996) Long-term follow-up of indolent mastocytosis in adults. J Int Med 239:157-164
Langer K, Wolff K (1990) Das klinische Spektrum der Mastozytosen. Hautarzt 41:188-195
Lennert K (1962) Zur pathologischen Anatomie von Urticaria pigmentosa und Mastzellenretikulose. Klin Wschr 40:61-67
Lennert K, Parwaresch MR (1979) Mast cells and mast cell neoplasia. Histopathology 3:339
Lippert U, Henz BM (1996) Long-term effect of interferon alpha treatment in mastocytosis. Br J Dermatol 134:1164-1165
Longley BJ, Morganroth GS, Tyrell BA (1993) Altered metabolism of mast cell growth factor (c-kit ligand) in cutaneous mastocytosis. N Engl J Med 328:1302-1307
Longley JB, Tyrrell L, Lu S-Z, Ma Y-S, Langley K, Ding T, Duffy T, Jacobs P, Tang LH, Modlin I (1996) Somatic c-kit activating mutation in urticaria pigmentosa and aggressive mastocytosis: establishment of clonality in a human mast cell neoplasm. Nature Genetics 121:312-314

Metcalfe DD (1991) Classification and diagnosis of mastocytosis; current status. J Invest Dermatol 96:2 S–4 S
Nagata H, Worobec AS, Oh CK, Chowdhury BA, Tannenbaum S, Suzuki Y, Metcalfe DD (1995) Identification of a point mutation in the catalytic domain of the protooncogene c-kit in peripheral blood mononuclear cells of patients who have mastocytosis with an associated dermatologic disorder. Proc Natl Acad Sci USA 92:10560–10564
Parks A, Camisa C (1988) Reddish-brown macules with teleangiectasia and pruritus. Urticaria pigmentosa-teleangiectasia macularis eruptiva perstans (TMEP) variant, with systemic mastocytosis. Arch Dermatol 124:429–433
Roberts LJ, Sweetman BJ, Lewis RA, Austen KF, Oates JA (1980) Increased production of prostaglandin D_2 in patients with systemic mastocytosis. New Engl J Med 303:1400–1404
Robinson HM Jr, Kile RL, Hitch JM, Raleigh NC, Robinson RCV (1962) Bullous urticaria pigmentosa. Arch Dermatol 85:346–354
Rodermund OE, Biersack HJ, Rohner HG (1978) Szintigraphische Veränderungen an Leber und Milz bei Urticaria pigmentosa. Hautarzt 29:478–480
Sagher F, Even-Paz Z (1967) Mastocytosis and the mast cell. Karger, Basel-New York
Soter NA, Austen KF, Wasserman SI (1979) Oral sodium cromoglycate in the treatment of systemic mastocytosis. N Engl J Med 301:465–469
Stege H, Schöpf E, Ruzicka T, Krutmann J (1996) High-dose UVA1 for urticaria pigmentosa. Lancet 347:64
Taylor G, Wojnarowska F, Chia Y, Kennedy C (1993) Treatment of urticaria pigmentosa by corticosteroids applied under a hydrocolloid dressing. Eur J Dermatol 3:276–278
Travis WD, Li CY, Bergstrahl EJ, Yam LT, Swee RG (1988) Systemic mast cell disease, analysis of 58 cases and literature review. Medicine 67:345–368
Unna PG (1887) Beiträge zur Anatomie und Pathogenese der Urtikaria simplex und pigmentosa. Dermatol Studien H3, Voss, Hamburg Leipzig
Webb TA, Lai CH, Lung TY (1982) Systemic mast cell disease: A clinical and hematopathologic study of 26 cases. Cancer 49:927–938
Worobec AS, Kirshenbaum AS, Schwartz LB, Metcalfe DD (1996) Treatment of three patients with systemic mastocytosis with interferon alpha-2b. Leukemia and Lymphoma 22: 501–508

10 Diagnosis of Urticaria

T. Zuberbier and B. M. Henz

10.1 Practical Approach

A search for the causes of urticaria is regarded an unsurmountable task by some physicians since it seems to be time consuming, rarely successful, and accordingly frustrating. The general principles of diagnosis, as outlined here, are to provide simple guidelines for a straight forward and logical diagnostic approach. For the diagnosis of specific types of urticaria, the reader is referred to the respective chapters of this book where these are discussed more extensively and in greater detail.

Of all diagnostic procedures outlined below, a thorough history is the most important measure, since positive skin tests and even the detection of specific serum IgE may be clinically irrelevant for diverse reasons (Pastorello 1995; Bernhisel-Broadbeut 1992). Further diagnostic procedures should be selected, dependent on the suspicions elicited by the meticulous history.

Diagnostic Procedure in Patients with Urticaria

A. Basic diagnostic measures:
   1. Patient history (see questionnaire, Appendix A)
   2. Physical examination
   3. Laboratory tests (routine CBC and diff.)
   4. Patient diary (often very helpful)

B. Narrowing down of possible eliciting factors by:
   1. Temporary avoidance of possible causes (e.g. drugs, food; see Appendix D)
   2. Therapeutic elimination of possible causes

C. Confirmation of possible diagnosis by:
   1. Provocation testing
      a) Physical tests (pressure, cold etc.)
      b) Physical exercises (cholinergic urticaria)
      c) Oral, inhalative provocation
      d) Skin tests (prick test, intracutaneous test)

2. Further laboratory tests, as deemed appropriate:
   a) Cultures for bacteria (infections)
   b) Serology (for viral, bacterial and parasitic antibodies)
   c) Liver enzymes
   d) Autoantibodies, possibly cryoglobulins
   e) Complement + C1-INH level
   f) Specific + total IgE
   g) Serum electrophoresis
   h) Stool for candida, parasites
   i) Gastroscopy (helicobacter)
   j) Dental examination
3. Skin and bone marrow biopsy (vasculitis, mastocytosis)
4. X-rays (lung, sinuses)
5. Sonography of upper abdomen and lymph nodes

The first diagnostic step in urticaria must be the verification of urticarial reactions. This can be done with a few questions regarding the shape of the lesions, their distribution and duration, and the associated local and systemic symptoms, particularly itching. In case the patient has wheals at the time of his visit, their inspection is helpful in the diagnosis. A test for dermographism to rule out the frequently associated dermographic urticaria should be done at this point. This entire procedure can be done within 2–3 minutes.

Subsequently, a more thorough history should be done to identify possible causes. Since this requires at least 15 minutes, it is easier, more time saving and more effective to send the patient back into the waiting room with an extensive questionnaire about possible causes of urticaria (see Appendix A). Alternatively, the list of items given below should be discussed with the patient.

Items To Be Asked During a Thorough Patient History (the Questionnaire in Appendix A Can Be Used Instead)

1. Frequency and duration of urticaria
2. Diurnal variation
3. shape, size and distribution of wheals
4. Associated angioedema
5. Associated subjective symptoms
6. Family history regarding urticaria, atopy
7. Previous or currently existing allergies, infections, internal diseases or other possible causes
8. Induction by physical agents
9. Use of drugs (including injections, immunizations and home remedies)
10. Food intolerance

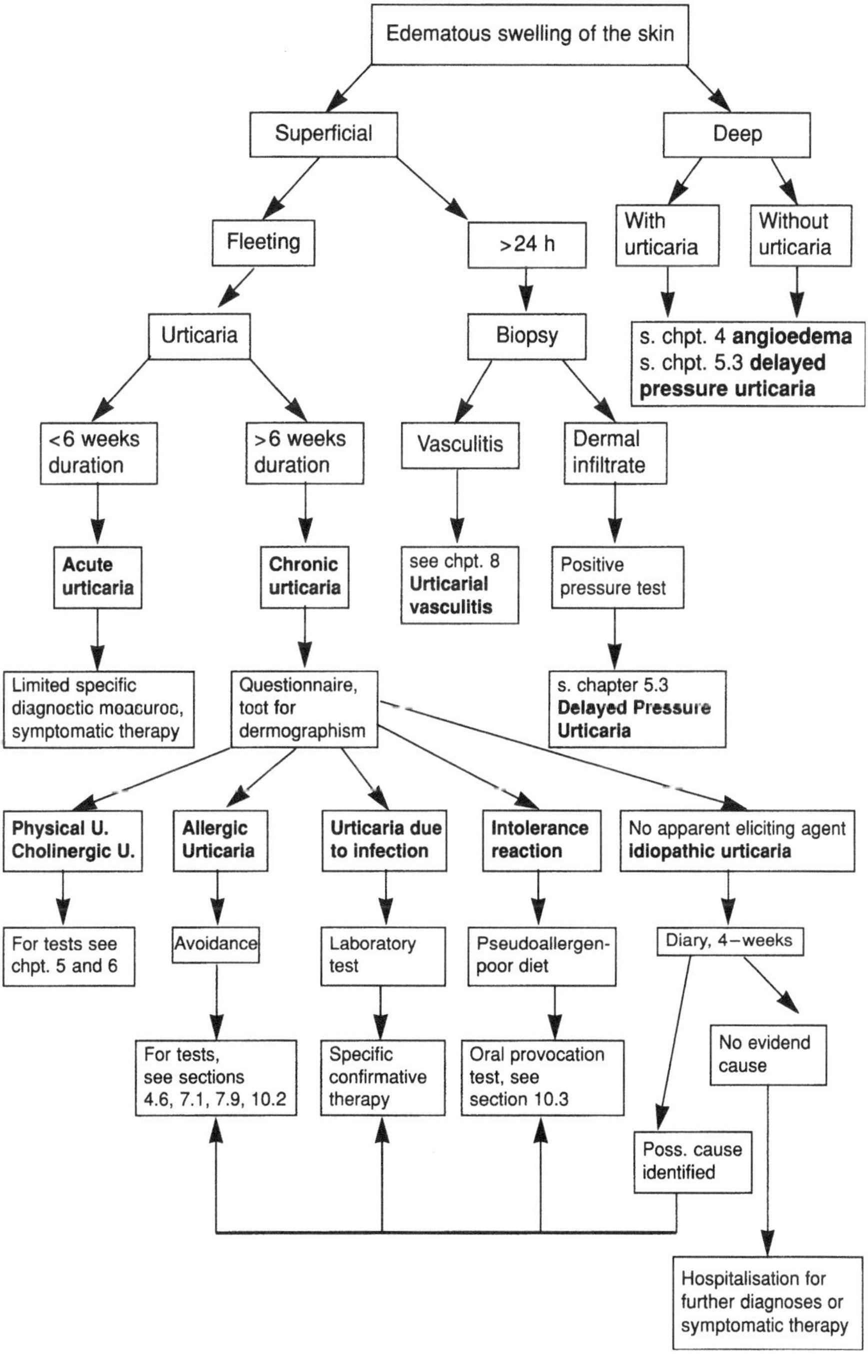

Fig. 10.1. Flow sheet as an aide in the stepwise procedure for the diagnosis of urticaria

11. Smoking habits
12. Type of work
13. Hobbies
14. Occurrence in relation to weekends, holidays and foreign travel
15. Surgical or other implantations
16. Reactions to insect stings
17. Relationship to the menstrual cycle
18. Response to therapy

When a special type of urticaria is suspected by history, the diagnosis should be confirmed by provocation tests. Furthermore, specific laboratory tests should be done as indicated. These yield positive results in maximally 20% of patients. Routine laboratory tests are not worthwhile and uneconomical (Table 10.1), particularly since positive results are rarely causally related to the urticaria.

As a further outpatient measure, the patient can be asked to keep a diary (see Appendix B). His notes often yield additional information and hints about possible causes, particularly after he has been educated about potential eliciting factors during his discussion with the physician. If allergy or an intolerance to a drug are suspected, this specific preparation should be omitted and replaced by a drug from a different chemical class if necessary. Subsequent amelioration or remission supports the suspected diagnosis. Reexposure to the suspected drug is usually not necessary, in view of the potentially dangerous reactions. When an allergy or intolerance to food instead of drugs is suspected, the same procedures should be followed. Even if the likelihood of success seems low on the basis of the medical history, a trial with a low-pseudoallergen diet (see Chapter 11 and Appendix D) is worthwhile in view of

Table 10.1. Positive laboratory tests in patients with acute and chronic urticaria irrespective of their pathogenetic significance (Kraig et al. 1980; Stemmler and Lischken 1979; Doeglas 1975; Zuberbier et al. 1995). Causal relation ship is rare, a screening is not indicated

Result	Frequency [%]
Positive stool for candida	9–21
Sinusitis and tonsillitis	0–17
Dental problems	0–16
C3 + C4	1–14
Thyroid antibodies	9
Urinary changes	3.5
Cryoglobulins	3
Helicobacter pylori	1–2
ANA	1–2
ESR	1
Eosinophilia	0–2
Worm eggs or parasites in the stool	0–1
RF ($\geq$1:10)	0
Specific IgE for candida	0

the fact that in some studies, more than 70% of patients with chronic urticaria derive benefit from it (Zuberbier et al. 1995; Haustein 1996; see also Chapters 2 and 3). A number of the patients are not aware of the possible associations.

Oral or other systemic provocation tests should generally be done only on hospitalized patients. This holds particularly for provocation tests with drugs. Patients should be free of symptoms prior to testing. Since this is not always possible, even with hospitalized patients, an exposure can be tried under close observation of the patient for worsening of symptoms, since the tested agent may be an aggravating factor of the basic urticarial symptomatology (Wüthrich 1983). In our hands, the symptomatology in these reactions is however rarely reproducible and relates instead to the level of expectation of the patient (own unpublished observation). Another possible reason is that the original reactions were pharmacological and due to higher doses or excitement of the patient during e.g. surgical procedures with local anestethics, so that the symptoms are not reproducible during testing with ordinary doses.

If hospitalization is possible and feasible, this is of advantage since the patient can be tested away from his daily environment and from the eliciting stimuli operative under these conditions. In all patients suspected to suffer from food-induced urticaria, it is worthwhile to order a minimal diet con-

Table 10.2. Special examinations only to be performed, in addition to CBC, differential and ESR, in case of a specific suspected cause of urticaria (not for screening)

Type I allergy	Infections	Infestations
Skin tests	Cultures	CBC and diff.
Total IgE	Serology (mononucleosis)	Total IgE
Specific IgE	Liver enzymes	Stool for worm eggs/ parasites
CBC and diff.	Sonography, upper abdomen	Serology
Omissions of e.g. food, drugs	Sinuses	Sonography, upper abdomen
Provocation tests	Dental status	
	Gastroscopy	
Malignant diseases	**Autoimmune diseases (see also Chapter 8)**	**Hormonal disturbances**
CH50	RF	T3, T4
C3, C4, C1q	Antinuclear antibodies	Thyroid antibodies
C1 INH	Circulating immune complexes	Ca, P
Protein electrophoresis	Anti-IgE	
CEA	CH50	
X-rays	C3, C4	
Sonography	Immunohistology	
Bone marrow biopsy		

sisting of potatoes, rice and water at the beginning of hospitalization. This excludes with high probability type I allergy against food as causative factor, since in type I allergy, in contrast to pseudoallergy, symptoms cease soon after allergen avoidance. A low-pseudoallergen diet or an elimination diet can be instituted thereafter (see Chapter 11 and Appendix D).

10.2 Tests for Allergy

10.2.1 General Aspects

If allergic causes of urticaria are suspected by history, specific tests with the suspected substance should be done. Although in type I allergy, skin and in vitro tests are possible, double blind placebo controlled in vivo provocation tests are currently thought to be the gold standard for detecting a relevant type-I-allergy (Pastorello 1995), and they are the only possibility for testing in case of pseudoallergies (see Section 10.2.3). Preferentially, the same route and circumstances under which the suspected agent gained entrance into the body, should be used for testing. When performing skin tests, it should be remembered that these have sometimes a low sensitivity in food allergy and that they are invalid for all types of pseudoallergens (see Section 10.2.3).

Veritable type I allergies are found particularly often in chronic intermittent urticaria, and they are only of minor importance in chronic continuous and in acute urticaria.

10.2.2 Skin Tests for Type I Allergies

Skin tests for mast cell-dependent type I allergic urticaria can be done using 5 different methods.

Prick tests are used very commonly because of their simplicity. The test is done by placing a drop of the allergen extract on the skin and pressing the tip of a lancet at an angle of 45-90° centrally about 1 mm through the epidermis, avoiding any type of bleeding. In this way, about 3 μl of the solution enter the skin (Fig. 10.2). In case of natural foods, the testing can be performed by first pricking the food and then using this lancet for pricking the skin.

For *scratch testing*, the skin is longitudinal scratched with a lancet or a needle (Fig. 10.3) or an area of about 1 cm^2 is superficially scratched, and a drop of the allergen extract or the raw test material is then applied to this area.

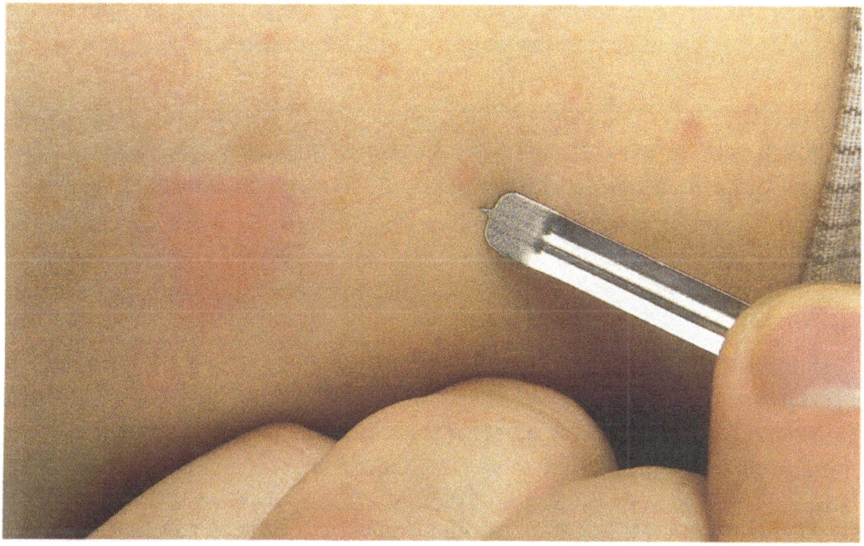

Fig. 10.2. Prick test with a positive reaction to walnut extracts (*on the left*) and two negative reactions to other allergens. The lancet is pressed through a drop of the test reagent into the skin

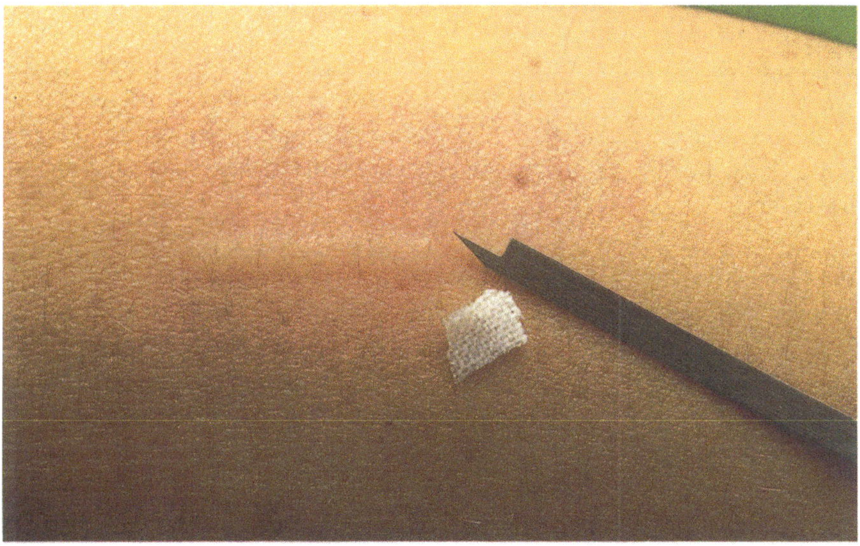

Fig. 10.3. Scratch test with whealing reaction in response to histamine. The skin was linearly scratched with a lancet, and the test solution was thereafter applied to the site on a small cotton pad

During *intracutaneous testing*, about 20 µl of the sterile extract in a tuberculin syringe are slowly injected intradermally with a fine needle (30 gauge).

The *rubbing test* is done prior to other types of skin tests primarily for safety reasons in patients who are suspected to be highly sensitized. It can also been done with raw material, as in the prick and scratch tests. Wheals appear preferentially around hair follicles since penetration at these sites is best. Readings are done after 20 minutes. The test is 10000 times less sensitive than intracutaneous tests and 100 times less sensitive than prick and scratch tests.

All tests are done on the upper or lower arm for safety reasons since in case of severe reactions, a tourniquet can be applied. When tests are done on the far more sensitive back, the test substances should first be pretested on the arm with a prick test for safety reasons. The distance between individual test sites should be at least 3 cm, preferably 5 cm, in order to avoid an influence of one test site on the other or to allow for exact evaluation of individual sites in case of very large reactions.

During all tests, controls should be done with the vehicle (negative control) as well as with histamine as positive control (0.01% solution for intracutaneous tests and 0.1% solution for prick tests, or diluted 1:10000 and 1:1000, respectively).

Tests are read after 15–20 minutes and if possible also again after 6–8 hours, the latter to detect late phase IgE-mediated reactions. Normal histamine wheals should be 4–6 mm in diameter for prick tests and 12–16 mm for intracutaneous tests. Whealing reactions in response to allergens are quantified in relation to the histamine wheal, i.e. 2+ at equal size, 3+ when the reaction is larger and 1+ when it is half the size of the histamine wheal. Very large wheals or pseudopodia are classified as 4+. A more exact quantification can be done by planimetry or by measuring the product of the diameters at right angles, divided by 2.

The *epicutaneous test* is done exclusively to rule out contact urticaria (see Chapter 7). It may also be used to confirm a positive prick test. Patch tests are done as for contact eczema. Readings are done after 20–60 minutes and again at 8 hours for the detection of possible delayed urticarial reactions (see Chapter 7). Since the intact skin is impermeable to many substances, penetration of the allergen can be enhanced by rubbing the skin with a firm agent (*rubbing test*).

There are only a few contraindications to skin testing (see below). Furthermore, one should consider that the skin reactivity is influenced by many factors (see below). This, it is of paramount importance to stop H_1-antihistamine treatment at least 2–3 days prior to testing and for several weeks for long acting preparations like astemizole. Sympathomimetics should be stopped one day before testing. Tranquillizers, tricyclic antidepressants and neuroleptics with H_1-blocking activity should be allowed an appropriate wash-out time as well. Corticosteroids at low doses (up to 40 mg) and after a one-week treatment are not contraindicated, but data regarding higher doses and longer therapy are not available. Many other antiallergic and antiinflammatory drugs like disodiumcromoglycate, theophyllin, aspirin or H_2-blockers have no influence on testing. Skin tests can also be done without special precautions during childhood.

Contraindications to Skin Testings (in Parenthesis: Possible Exceptions)

- Severe systemic diseases like pneumonia, decompensated cardiac insufficiency
- Pregnancy (relative contraindication)
- Thrombocytopenia (possibly for intracutaneous tests)
- Defects of coagulation, possibly for intracutaneous tests (not during coumarin treatment)
- Acute allergic symptoms (not with inhalation allergies)
- Impetigo
- Extensive cutaneous inflammation

Factors Influencing Reactions to Prick- Scratch- and Intracutaneous Tests (for Positive and for Negative Influences)

- Quantity of allergens
- Reactivity of mast cells
- Reactivity of the target tissue
- Depth of injection
- Body region (↑ on the upper back)
- Time of day (↑ in the evening)
- Menstruation cycle (↑ prior to mensis)
- Age (↑ during the 3. decade)
- Associated diseases (↑ with dermographic urticaria, ↓ with ichthyosis and atopic eczema)
- immunotherapy (↓)
- Refractory period after whealing reaction or anaphylaxis (↓)
- H1-type antihistamines (↓)
- Psychotrophic drugs with H1-type antihistamine activity (↓)
- Sympathomimetics (↓)

Positive skin tests have been found on routine testing in 2–8% of patients for pollen and house dust mite, although the patients had no corresponding symptoms. The same holds for fish antigens (Bernhisel-Broadbent et al. 1992). The allergens must thus be considered as clinically irrelevant. These patients may however develop symptoms at a later time point. This is particularly observed with allergens that are chemically related or that crossreact immunologically. Prominent examples are the profilins which are ubiquitously distributed in the vegetable kingdom, tropomyosin in insects, crustacians and mites, or carbohydrates in otherwise unrelated substances (Pastorello 1995). Development of tolerance, as observed e.g. in children with milk allergy after 2–3 years, is another reason why skin tests continue to be positive.

False-positive skin tests are caused by vasoactive amines, histamine liberators or toxic agents, as observed in insect or plant extracts, but also in food extracts or drugs. These substances can also increase reactions that are otherwise only subclinically positive. The coexistence of dermographic urticaria is another reason for false-positive reactions.

False-negative reactions are usually observed after incorrect application of allergens or when the patient has taken antihistamines. A further cause is the lack of specific allergens relevant for the patients in the commercial test extract. Allergen extracts are also less stable after dilution, particularly extracts from fruits and vegetables. Adding more glycerin for stabilization is on the other hand problematic since it can increase the number of false-positive reactions. In case of suspected false-negative reactions, it is recommendable to use fresh substances for testing. Even in this case, a negative test result need not rule out the type-I allergy since some allergens only originate within the body due to pH-changes or reactions of enzymes. As a final possible cause for false-negative reactions, the refractory period after massive generalized whealing reactions or anaphylactic reactions, e.g. after massive insect sting reactions, should be considered. In this case, tests should be done only 2–3 weeks later. Under normal conditions, testing for type I allergies can however be done at weekly intervals at the same test site with reproducible results (Grabbe et al. 1993).

10.2.3 Provocation Tests for Type-I Allergies

Because of their limited use and the unreliability of skin tests in a broad range of circumstances, oral or parenteral provocation tests with the suspected agents are unavoidable for the diagnosis of urticaria (Pastorello 1995). These should be done using the usual precautionary measures. Suspected drugs need not be tested when the history is clear and when alternative agents are available. In case of suspected pseudoallergy to local anesthetics, pain medication or antibiotics, provocation tests with alternative substances via the same route are however frequently indicated in order to rule out reactivity to these agents and for reassurance of the patient.

Oral provocation with food can even be done in small children. Dependent on the history, the substances are generally given in a raw or cooked state for blinded testing. The taste and the appearance of the food should be changed in order to give the patients no clues as to their nature. The real situation during ordinary exposure can e.g. also be mimicked by the same processing of the food and by adding alcoholic beverages. Since the amount of the allergen may also be of importance, a strict exposure test scheme should be followed, as outlined below. The patient should always be symptom-free at the start of the provocation testing. If instead, exacerbations of preexisting mild whealing is chosen as a diagnostic criterion, results are mostly confusing and uninterpretable.

Stepwise Provocation Diet for Type-I Allergy Testing

Step 1 *Milk and eggs:*
cheese, yoghurt, cottage cheese, milk, eggs, butter, salt, onions.
No fruits!

Step 2 *Carbohydrates and fruits:*
bread, baked goods, pudding, honey, marmalade,
fruit juices, tomatoes, celery, fresh fruits

Step 3 *Meat and sausages:*
bacon, beef, pork, chicken.
No tinned meat or sausages

Step 4 *Fish and crustaceans:*
fish in tins, sardines,
cooked or fried fish, marinade herring, crabs

Step 5 *Full exposure test:*
normal breakfast and lunch.
Dinner: e.g. ox-tail soup, crabs with mayonnaise, meat with sauces,
potato dumplings, sauerkraut, fruits with whipped cream,
red or white wine, coffee

If food allergy is suspected without clear indications regarding the nature of the allergen, the patient can first be given a minimal diet consisting of potatoes, rice and water until all symptoms have abated. Then a stepwise daily provocation meal, as shown above. In this way, one can often identify the eliciting substance within 1–2 weeks in hospital and in close cooperation with the dietitian. Such procedure also helps to allay the patient's fears and his unnecessary avoidance of numerous innocuous foods. In very cooperative patients, this procedure can also be done on an ambulatory basis. Patients are told in this case to maintain a bland diet, adding a suspected substance every 2–3 days, until they can eat normally. In case of intercurring reactions, the suspected substance must be avoided for a while; it can then be retested later on to confirm the diagnosis. In children with milk or other types of food allergy, one should proceed as follows:

Diet in Toddlers and Babies with Food Allergies

1. History, diary for 2 weeks
2. Elimination of suspicious agents
3. Elimination diet:
   ≤3 months: human milk, casein hydrolysate
   3–6 months: add rice, cereals
   6–24 months: add vitamins, carrots, apple sauce, pears, pumpkin, lamb
4. Normal diet, adding new types of food every 4 days

One must of course make sure that the suspected food intolerance is not due to other causes like pyloric stenosis. In children with a high risk of atopy, cow's milk should be avoided during breast feeding. These children should be either breast fed for the first 6 months or given casein hydrolysates, with addition of other types of food only after 6 months. Citrus fruits and wheat should be avoided until the end of the first year of life, eggs, nuts and fish until the end of the second year of life.

10.2.4
Laboratory Tests for Type-I Allergies

Measurement of total serum-IgE serves only as an orientation during the diagnostic work-up for type-I allergies. Elevations indicate a predisposition to atopy or other types of diseases associated with elevated serum-IgE like parasitic diseases, bullous pemphigoid or mycosis fungoides. In up to 90% of patients with type-I food allergy, total serum IgE is elevated. Specific IgE determinations are too expensive for screening but are of value when skin tests cannot be done or when these results are incongruent with the clinical history.

The basic concept for the procedure of specific RAST-tests are shown in Fig. 10.4. This test is curently used with a number of modifications, particularly because the use of radio-nucleotides is preferably avoided. The basic results are however unchanged.

Disadvantages of this test are its high cost and the limited number of allergens that can be tested. Furthermore, problems with the instability of allergens exist, as described above for prick tests. Determinations of specific IgE against fruits and vegetables can therefore not be recommended. Some commercial

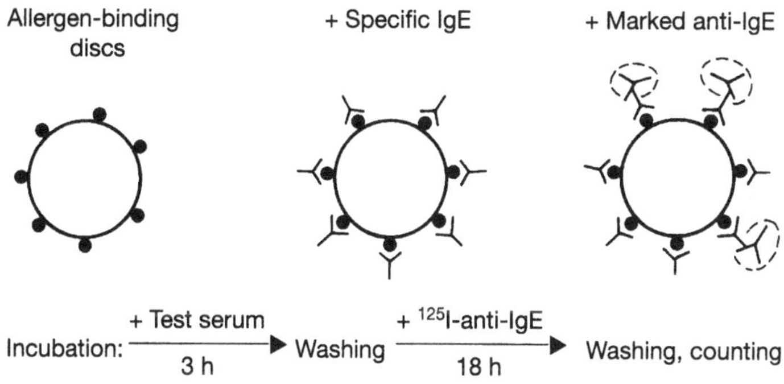

Fig. 10.4. Scheme for the methodology of the original RAST method

laboratories perform a broad spectrum of tests for IgG against food allergens. Since such antibodies are made by the body against many foods and since they have no pathological significance, such tests are not recommended, particularly since the results tend to confuse the patients. So-called cytotoxic tests are similarly without diagnostic value.

In vitro tests studying histamine release from blood basophils in the presence of the allergens in question are on the other hand reliable, but rather laborious. The so-called basophil degranulation test which is done after counting basophils in blood before and after in vitro addition of allergens, has also received no general acceptance. Lymphocytc transformation tests are not reliable for the diagnosis of urticarial drug reactions.

10.3 Diagnosis of Intolerance Reactions

As mentioned before, pseudoallergic intolerance reactions are a frequent underlying cause of chronic urticaria and drug-induced urticaria. As with other types of intolerance, a good history is of paramount importance for the proper diagnosis. This is generally easy when the eliciting agent, e.g. an analgesic drug, has caused intense and acute reactions. The cause is less evident in delayed reactions and particularly in chronic types of the disease. There is for example only a low correlation between the patient history and proven aspirin intolerance on provocation test in patients with chronic recurrent urticaria. Possible reasons for this are multiple:

- Patients may wrongly interpret symptoms as disease-related.
- Reactions are only elicited under additive or enhancing circumstances: e.g. during viral infections, when aspirin or preservative-rich food are taken together or when the patients also drink alcohol.

- The contents of naturally occurring food ingredients, e.g. salicylates or parahydroxybenzoic acid in fruits, are highly variable, so that reactions fail to occur regularly on exposure to the same agent.
- The patient has reacted clinically very recently and is in a refractory period at the time of testing. If this is suspected, provocation should be repeated after a few days.
- Spontaneous remission has occurred (in 50% of patients with ASA intolerance within one year).

Despite all these difficulties, a thorough history of afflicted patients generally provides valuable clues. Its efficacy can be markedly improved using standardized questionnaires which the patient can fill in while waiting in the office or at home (Appendix A). It is also helpful to have the patient fill in a diary for 2–4 weeks (Appendix B). Since a combination of different eliciting agents can be responsible, the diary should be as exact as possible, and since the symptoms recorded by the patient can be very diffuse and nonspecific, those typically observed during intolerance reactions are summarized in Table 10.3.

Unfortunately, there are currently no reliable skin or in vitro tests available for intolerance reactions, in contrast to IgE-mediated allergies. Suspected agents on history must therefore be confirmed by provocation tests.

All provocation tests should be done during hospitalization, for safety reasons. Drugs as well as other agents that have caused acute or severe reactions should always be tested with an indwelling intravenous catheter and with readily available first aid medication. During drug testing, one should only do provocation tests with the suspected agent when further treatment is urgently needed. In all other cases, so-called negative provocation tests with alternative substances should be done. Particularly for analgesics and local anesthetics, an abundance of alternative preparations are available, so that the

Table 10.3. Objective and subjective symptoms during intolerance reactions

Objective symptoms	Subjective symptoms
Urticaria/whealing	Tingling
Erythema (particularly on face and chest)	Itching
Angioedema	Headache
Hoarseness	Palpitations
Swelling of the nasal mucosa	Shortness of breath
Sneezing	Flushing
Tearing of the eyes	Sweating
Bronchospasm	Abdominal pain
Diarrhea	Nausea
Fever	Dazedness
Syncope	Dizziness

risk of an anaphylactic reaction on reexposure is avoided. If a preservative or another additive in drugs is suspected, one may expose the specific components under the precautionary measures mentioned.

Hospitalization during testing is not only advantageous for safety reasons, but also for standardization of the procedure. Freedom from symptoms is an essential prerequisite for provocation tests. For this purpose, patients with suspected food intolerance should be on a potato-rice-diet for at least 3 days. Some physicians initially give a laxative in order to remove potential eliciting or sustaining stimuli from the intestines. When the patient is free of symptoms, he should be switched to a low-pseudoallergen diet (see Section 11.2.2.1 and Appendix D1), and testing should be started. Pseudoallergens are either additives (dyes, preservatives, antioxidants) or naturally occurring components in food (e.g. salicylates, parahydroxybenzoic acid). A scheme for testing the most frequent eliciting agents of intolerance reactions in food is given below. In individual cases, suspected agents, e.g. sweeteners, can be added to this list.

Compared with the frequency of reactions to pseudoallergen-rich food, positive reactions on testing encapsulated individual pseudoallergens is low in patients with chronic urticaria (<20%, Zuberbier et al. 1995). Such testing is furthermore time consuming. The reasons for the low sensitivity of the test are more likely due to not as yet identified pseudoallergens in natural food (e.g. aromatic substances, according to recent own, unpublished data) which are more frequent causes of pseudoallergics.

As with skin tests, provocation tests should also be done in the absence of agents that might support or suppress the symptomatology. Thus, all suspected eliciting drugs should be stopped prior to testing or, if necesssary, treatment must be continued with alternative drugs from different chemical groups. Depending on the previous dose, antihistamines and corticosteroids can generally be discontinued 3 days before testing, although 3 weeks may be necessary after high dose, prolonged steroid therapy. An exception to this rule is astemizole because of its very long half-life. The time of about 30 days needed for elimination of the drug may be bridged by suppressing the patient's symptoms with ordinary antihistamines that have a short half-life.

β-Blockers should be stopped before testing since in case of anaphylactic shock, the effect of adrenaline is blocked.

Provocation tests should approximate as closely as possible the natural exposure to the suspected substances. In most cases, this means oral provocation. Ideally, the substance should be given in a bland capsule and under double-blind, placebo controlled conditions. Principally, only one substance or one group of substances should be exposed per day. In case of a reaction, testing must be stopped for one or even 2–3 days because of the refractory period. Placebo testing can however be done during that time. Preferably, the substance that is suspected most should be tested at the end of the test period or before a weekend.

Protocol for Provocation Tests of Known Pseudoallergens in Patients with Food-Induced Intolerance (Not for Explorative Purposes)

The following agents should be filled into colorless gelatin capsules.

A) Coloring mixture: chinolin yellow, yellow orange S, azorubin, amaranth, erythrosine, ponceau red, patent blue, indigotin, brilliant black, ferric III oxide red, cochenille, *5 mg each*
B1) Sorbic acid, 500 mg
B2) Sodium benzoate, parahydroxybenzoic acid, 500 mg each
B3) Sodium metabisulfite, 50 mg
C) Sodium nitrate, 100 mg, sodium glutamate, 200 mg
D) Placebo: lactose
E) Tartrazin, 50 mg
F) Salicylic acid, 150 mg
G) BHA (butyl hydroxy anisole), propylgallate BHT (butyl hydroxy toluol), tocopherol, 50 mg each

- To exclude pseudoallergy against additives a combination af all capsules can be given at one time. If a positive reaction is observed, one group each has to be given on a daily basis.
- After each positive reaction, no further testing should be done for at least one day (except possibly placebo). Positive reactions should be verified by reexposure on some other day.

Special note: There is evidence for additional, as yet unidentified pseudo-allergens in natural food which appear to be responsible for the majority of reactions. The test as described above can therefore not be used as a screening test for pseudoallergies.

As with type-I allergies, intolerance reactions to food may have to be tested with the native foods. If at all possible, the patient should be exposed with the same food which is suspected to have caused his subsequent clinical reaction. There are several reasons for this:

- The same foods need not contain the same chemical components. This holds particularly for processed foods like baked goods, sweets etc. These products contain not only different declared additives from the respective producers, but the composition of certain products can change from batch to batch without the consumer being aware of this. Besides intolerance reactions, type-I allergic reactions to hidden allergens may also be involved. For example, chocolate frequently contains soy bean or peanut products which need not be declared and which are well-known type-I allergens. The same problem exists with natural products like vegetables since their contents e.g. salicylates, vary widely dependent on the type of vegetable, its ripeness and the region where it was grown.

- Many types of food cannot be given in an encapsulated form. As an alternative, they may be given mixed with puree or even be given via a stomach tube. During routine testing, this is of course a rather complicated procedure.
- If by history a combination of several foods is suspected, it may be meaningful to ask the patient to procure exactly the original food stuff for exposure in the reported combination. A number of intolerance reactions are not induced by single substances, but only by a combination of several factors. The most common example is the combination of low level stimuli together with alcoholic beverages.
- In case of bronchial reactions to beverages, evaporated molecules which are subsequently inhaled may be a cause. This has been proven for metabisulfite which may be added to refreshing beverages as preservatives. In a watery solution, particularly the presence of citric acid, as occurs e.g. in fruit juices, irritating SO_2 is generated. The air above a glass of orange may contain 1 ppm SO_2 and may thus induce bronchial reactions. 11% of asthmatics give a history of reactions to certain refreshing beverages.

Intramuscular injections represent an exception to the postulate to perform provocation tests along the normal way of application of a substance. In this case, the risk of difficult to treat, long lasting reactions is too great so that on principle, no i.m. provocation test should be done.

Protocol for Testing Local Anesthetics

- Testing of alternative substances if possible
- Never test substances that caused life-threatening reactions on history
- Test only with an indwelling intravenous catheter (with physiological saline)
- Have first aid medication at hand
- Follow always the testing sequence:
  1. Prick testing
  2. Intracutaneous testing
     In case 1 and 2 are negative, provocations can be done with slowly increasing doses.
  3. Subcutaneous injections at 30 minute intervals with 0.1 ml, 0.2 ml, 0.5 ml, 1 ml, 2 ml of test substance.

Analogously, subcutaneous and intravenous testing can be done with other drugs. Dosages must be chosen in dependence of the substance to be tested.

Prick and intracutaneous tests are negative in case of pseudoallergic reactions such as intolerance to local anesthetics, but they should always be done since in rare cases, type-I allergic reactions can coexist as well.

The following principle is important for testing local anesthetics: In case the reaction was life-threatening on history, the suspected substance should be tested only when it is therapeutically important. Otherwise, alternative preparations without additives which generally cause no reactions (e.g. lidocaine) should be tested and recommended for future treatments.

10.4 Other Laboratory Tests (Table 10.2)

Routine laboratory tests are of little value for the diagnosis of urticaria (see Table 10.1). The situation is different when specific underlying diseases are to be confirmed by laboratory tests (Table 10.2).

10.5 Differential Diagnosis

Wheals are clinically easy to identify because of their classical signs and symptoms (see Section 1.2). There are rarely difficulties to differentiate urticaria from other diseases. Problems arise only when the duration of individual wheals cannot be clearly defined or when itching is absent. Difficulties can exist when wheals are present together with other types of lesions, when they persist for a long time, such as in urticarial vasculitis, or when deep swellings are present, as in delayed pressure urticaria. In case of doubt, it is helpful to mark the edges of the wheals with a skin pen and to watch their evolution or resolution with time.

Differential Diagnosis of Acute and Chronic Urticaria

- Erythema multiforme
- Maculopapular rashes
- Erythema marginatum
- Erythema chronicum migrans
- Erythema anulare centrifugum
- Granuloma anulare
- Tinea corporis
- Sweet's syndrome

Erythema multiforme can at times be mistaken for urticaria when the typical target lesions (Fig. 10.5) or mucosal involvement are missing. Maculopapular rashes during drug reactions or viral infections can be easily distinguished

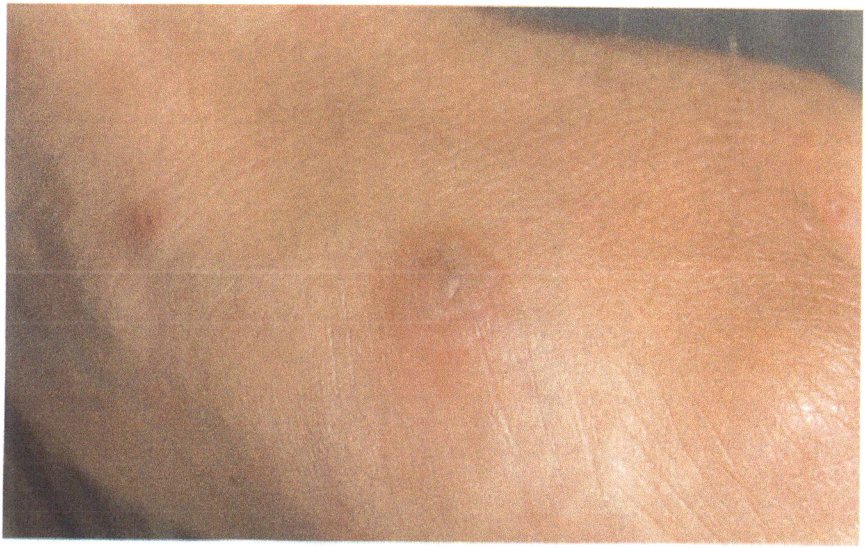

Fig. 10.5. Close-up of a typical target lesion in a patient with erythema multiforme. The center of the lesion is grayish in color, due to early blister formation

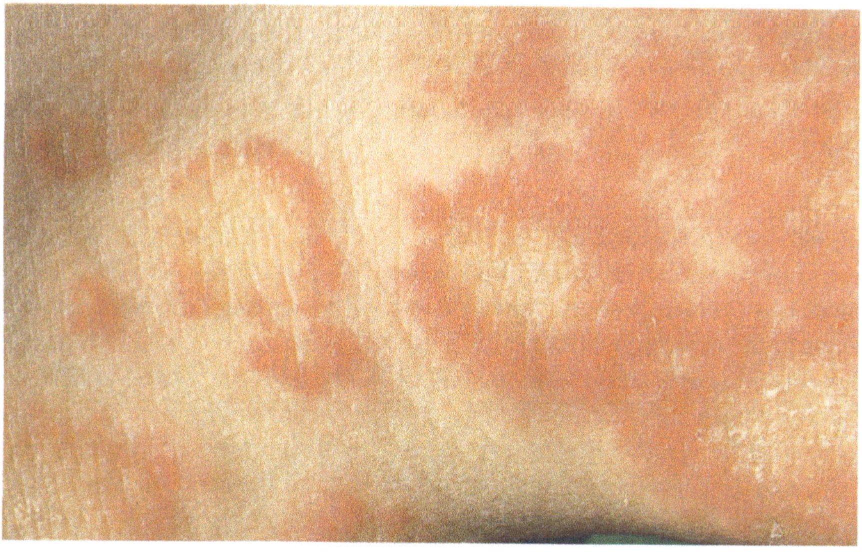

Fig. 10.6. Erythematous papules in an anular arrangement in a patient with bullous pemphigoid, prior to the development of blistering

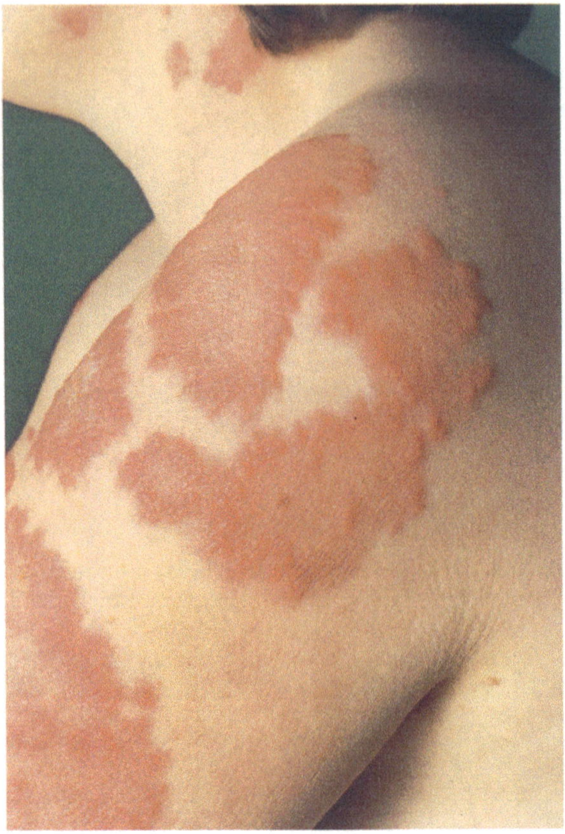

Fig. 10.7. Erythematous plaques studded with papules in a women with Sweet's syndrome. In contrast to wheals, the lesions persisted unchanged for several weeks

because of the persistence of the individual lesions and the residual purpuric component. Anular erythemas and rashes (see preceding overview) can be more of a problem, although they also persist longer than urticarial lesions. Prior to the development of typical blisters, bullous pemphigoid lesions can closely mimic urticarial reactions (Fig. 10.6). The lesions of Sweet's syndrome can represent a similar problem (Fig. 10.7), particularly since fever and leukocytosis can be a feature in some rare types of urticaria as well (see Sections 2.5, 5.3, 5.4). Tinea corporis lesions can be differentiated by their typical scaling.

Literature

Bernhisel-Broadbent J, Scanlon SM, Sampson HA (1992) Fish hypersensitivity. I. In vitro and oral challenge results in fish-allergic patients. J Allergy Clin Immunol 89:730–737

Cooper KD (1991) Urticaria and angioedema: Diagnosis and evaluation. J Am Acad Dermatol 25:166–176

Czarnetzki BM (1994) Neues zur Diagnostik und Therapie der Urtikaria. Allergologie 17: 2–5

Doeglas HMG (1975) Chronic urticaria. Clinical and pathogenetic studies on 141 patients. Dykstra Niemeyer, Groningen

Grabbe J, Zuberbier T, Wagenpfeil S, Czarnetzki BM (1993) Skin prick tests to common allergens in adult atopic eczema and rhinitis patients: Reproducibility on duplicate and repeated testing. Dermatology 186:113-117

Haustein U (1996) Pseudoallergen-free diet in the treatment of chronic urticaria. Acta Derm Venereol (Stockh) 76:498-499

Kraig M, Jacobson KW, Branch LB, Nelson HS (1980) Laboratory tests in chronic urticaria. JAMA 243:1644-1646

Pastorello EA (1995) Evaluating new tests for the diagnosis of food allergy. Allergy 50:289-291

Stemmler M, Lischka G (1979) Urticaria - reasonable diagnostic proceeding. Akt Dermatol 5:131-134

Wüthrich B (1983) Allergische und pseudoallergische Reaktionen der Haut durch Arzneimittel und Lebensmitteladditiva. Schweiz Rundschau Med (PRAXIS) 72:691-699

Zuberbier T, Czarnetzki BM (1995) Urtikaria - aktuelle Aspekte der Diagnostik und Therapie. Dtsch Dermatol 43:148-153

Zuberbier T, Chantraine-Hess S, Czarnetzki BM (1995) Pseudoallergen-free diet in the treatment of chronic urticaria - a prospective study. Acta Derm Venereol (Stockh) 75: 484-487

11 Urticaria Therapy

B.M. Henz, T. Zuberbier and E. Monroe

11.1 Basic Therapeutic Considerations

In contrast to the complex diagnostic approaches and procedures in urticaria, the therapy of most types of this disease is simple and logical (Fig. 11.1). After a thorough history and physical examination, three possible approaches can be followed:

- Avoidance of the eliciting stimulus is the most obvious and effective type of treatment since the direct cause of urticaria is removed and a cure can thus be achieved. Unfortunately, this type of treatment depends on the exact identification of the cause of urticaria which in turn can be very difficult. In IgE-dependent urticaria, it is, however, generally quite successful.
- The next best approach is aimed at the effector cell. Since very few drugs are effective at this level, it can be applied to only a limited extent.
- Currently, the most frequently used therapy acts at the level of the target tissue of mast cell mediators. Very effective drugs such as H_1 antihistamines (see below) are available for this purpose. They suppress the symptoms of urticaria and give the patient relief from the frequently vexing symp-

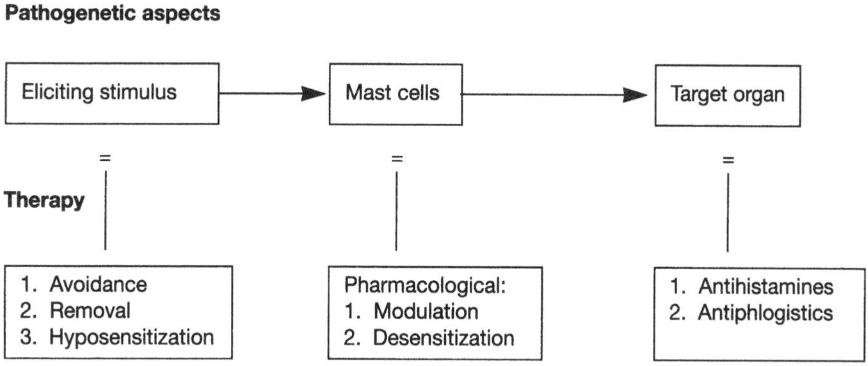

Fig. 11.1. Therapeutic principles in urticaria on the basis of its pathophysiology

tomatology. This holds for acute and chronic as well as for most types of physical urticaria dealt within different chapters of this book. Few types of urticaria (e.g. vasculitis, delayed pressure urticaria) can however not be effectively treated in this way, and the afflicted patients represent a therapeutic problem (see Section 11.4.2 for the treatment of special types of urticaria).

11.2 Treatment of Causes

With this therapeutic approach, diagnosis and treatment of urticaria are difficult to separate since a truly causative treatment requires a thorough diagnostic approach, resulting in the identification of the eliciting agent. A remission of urticaria after elimination of the suspected cause as well as provocation of the disease after reexposure provide final proof for the causative role of the elicitor. Treatment of the causes can be done by several approaches (Fig. 11.1).

11.2.1 Removal or Avoidance of the Cause

Whenever the eliciting factor of urticarial reactions can be eliminated, the situation is very simple. Examples are the surgical excision of implanted material or solid tumors or the prompt removal of the stinger after bee and wasp stings. If an acute urticaria is caused by the oral route, treatment with a laxative may be worthwhile to accelerate the excretion of the causative agent from the intestine. Care should however be taken in the choice of the laxative since those of plant origin are themselves a frequent cause of urticaria. Recently, prolonged remissions have been obtained in some severe cases of solar urticaria after plasmapheresis. In this situation, a causative serum factor has probably been removed.

Treatment of ongoing diseases which might cause or sustain chronic urticaria is imperative. Focal infections in the oral, the naso-pharyngeal or the gastrointestinal region should be treated appropriately, including elimination of helicobacter pylori or a massive candidosis. Parasites are to be eliminated with specific chemotherapeutic agents. For the treatment of lymphomas or autoimmune diseases, specific treatment should be initiated as far as available.

Far more frequently, the eliciting agent is not present within the body but is instead introduced from without. In these cases, a strategy of avoidance must be persued. This implies e.g. the discontinuation of drug treatment or a diet from which the suspected agent is eliminated. Once the cause is found, the patient should be advised regarding the choice of alternative drugs and the avoidance of crossreacting agents. In case of uncertainty, improvement of urticaria after discontinuation of treatment with the implicated drug, or the omission of certain foods or additives from the diet are an indirect proof for a possible causal relationship. If the patient suffers from physical urticaria, he should be instructed to avoid the eliciting factor as far as possible, e.g. he should not jump into cold water in case of cold urticaria. In patients with difficult to treat delayed pressure urticaria, the only solution may be a change of work (see Chapter 5).

Patients with urticaria should also be instructed to avoid aggravating factors. These include alcohol, a warm environment, viral infections, excessive physical exertion or often also aspirin which aggravates chronic urticaria in a sizable number of patients.

11.2.2 Dietary Management of Chronic Urticaria Due to Pseudoallergens

Once the diagnosis of pseudoallergy to food ingredients has been established in urticaria, a diet containing only low levels of pseudoallergens should be instituted and, if successful, be maintained for a prolonged period of time (at least 3–6 months) until spontaneous remission is achieved. In the past, avoidance of individual additives, as generally practiced, resulted in only minor or moderate success in the dietary management of urticaria patients (Juhlin 1981; Rudzki et al. 1980; Gibson and Clancy 1980), whereas responsiveness exceeding 70 % has been observed by Haustein (1996) and at our clinic in Berlin with a more restrictive diet (Zuberbier et al. 1995b) (see Table 11.1)

In the following section, a number of specific details and practical aspects of such a strict diet are described in cooperation with a dietician (I. Ehlers), and a summary of the diet is given in Appendix D, with some recipes in Appendix E. Recent unpublished results from our group suggest that aromatic residues in fruits like tomatoes and in wine cause positive reactions in up to 70% of our diet-responsive patients. The success of our diet may thus be due to the fact that a number of foods containing such aromas are avoided together with the previously implicated additives.

Table 11.1. Response to a low-pseudoallergen diet in 64 patients with severe chronic urticaria during hospitalization and follow-up (Zuberbier et al. 1995a)

Response to diet in hospital, (chronic continuous urticaria, no dermographic urticaria)	73.4%
Maintenance of response during 6 months follow-up	96.8 %

11.2.2.1 Practical Guidelines for the Dietary Avoidance of Pseudoallergens

I. EHLERS and T. ZUBERBIER

In the literature, a wide variety of diets, including a broad range of different foods, are proposed for the treatment of intolerance reactions to foods. Because of basic inconsistencies in the composition of these diets and unfavorable clinical experiences, we have developed a new diet in close cooperation with dieticians (see also Section 10.3 and Appendix D1). This diet has proven to be a highly effective means to treat pseudoallergic intolerance reactions to food (Zuberbier et al. 1995b). It prohibits all industrially processed foods which might contain additives like dyes, preservatives or antioxidants, and it lacks almost entirely histamine liberators which are commonly found in strawberries, fermented cheese, crustaceans, mollusks, nuts and shellfish. It contains however minor amounts of naturally occurring pseudoallergens like salicylates or parahydroxybenzoic acid in vegetables. Since the diet is not entirely devoid of pseudoallergens, we propose to call it "low-pseudoallergen diet", in contrast to the term "allergen-free diet" currently used in the literature. Since pseudoallergic reactions are dose-dependent, the low quantities of natural pseudoallergens and histamine liberators that are still consumed with the diet advocated by us, fail to elicit clinical reactions. The low-pseudoallergen diet has also proven to be practical in an outpatient setting although the patient makes more inadvertent mistakes in this situation. These mistakes can, however, readily be detected if the patient is instructed to carefully document his food intake in a diary.

The low-pseudoallergen diet should be maintained until freedom or improvement of symptoms is observed. In the majority of patients, symptoms abate already within seven days, although they may persist in 30–40% of patients for up to two weeks. In outpatients, improvement may therefore even take longer since an absolutely strict adherence to the diet is unlikely, and patients should be encouraged to maintain the diet initially for a longer period, i.e. for at least three weeks. The decrease of symptoms tends to run in waves, but despite these relapses, there is an overall decrease in intensity and frequency of urticaria with time. Reasons for relapse can at times be pinpointed to unintentional mistakes in the diet, the intake of analgesics, or to intercurrent viral infections. The patient should be informed about such potential pitfalls, so that his motivation is not adversely affected. In case improvement is not evident or only minor, a pseudoallergen-rich food should be eaten for one or two days which, if negative, will definitely rule out food intolerance as a cause of the urticaria. The possible coexistence of a type I allergy to specific foods should also be kept in mind and ruled out by appropriate testing (see Section 10.2). All in all, the initiation of the low-pseudoallergen diet can be accomplished in most patients on an outpatient basis, but with the occasional difficult patient, hospitalization may be the only means to clarify the diagnosis and to initiate effective dietary treatment.

Expanding the Diet

Once freedom of symptoms has been obtained with the diet, two possible further approaches can be chosen:

- The patient is hospitalized and undergoes double blind oral provocation testing, with additives in an encapsulated form, as outlined in Section 10.3. Thereafter or alternatively, a pseudoallergen-rich meal is given to verify the diagnosis. A subsequent stepwise addition of different foods to expand the diet can be instituted thereafter on an outpatient basis. Initially, only those foods should be introduced that rarely cause urticaria (Appendix D2). On choosing the sequence of added new food ingredients, the patient's history and his personal preferences should be taken into account.
- If hospitalization is not feasible the patient is further followed on an outpatient basis, without specific provocation tests, and the diet is expanded as described above.

Several specific points should be heeded during diet expansion: New types of food should be added at most every third day, since clinical reactions occur for up to 24 h after food intake in 50% of patients. These symptoms also need time to abate, and a subsequent refractory period might yield false negative results on rapidly instituted further testing. When symptoms recur, the newly added food should be avoided for several subsequent weeks, and the previously tolerated diet should be maintained until freedom of symptoms is obtained again. Other food ingredients can then be added using the same procedure. It is advisable to repeat testing of food that caused reactions earlier, after an extended period of remission in order to confirm that the specific substance was the cause for the relapse. This repeated testing is also valuable in view of the fact that reactivity to some substances is lost with time. Repeated provocation test should ideally be done in a blinded fashion in order to exclude psychological factors which might contribute to the patient's symptoms.

When expanding the diet, additive effects of several provoking agents should also be taken into account. It may thus be possible that each newly introduced food is tolerated without problems by itself, but that a combination of different food items induces a reaction.

The procedure, as outlined above, is generally well accepted by the patients, particularly since most of them appreciate the active involvement in their treatment. Patient compliance is generally better in patients whose symptoms were initially severe. Regular counseling of the patient by his physician and/or dietician is essential particularly during the initial weeks of therapy. The availability of recipes (examples, see Appendix E) is generally highly appreciated. If individual patients can however not be motivated sufficiently, a less stringent diet, supported by regular intake of antihistamines is preferable to a symptomatic treatment with antihistamines alone, particularly since avoidance of pseudoallergens probably favors the induction of remissions.

A few practical hints may be useful to avoid pitfalls in keeping the diet. Thus, industrially processed food may contain a number of further additives, e.g. for the purpose of prolonging its stability or in order to enhance it attractiveness. In Europe, each additive must be declared on the package, giving its name, group name or E-number. A few exceptions to this rule can be particularly problematic for highly sensitive patients. Thus, sulfur-containing products need to be declared in some countries only when the sulfur dioxide contents exceed 50 mg/kg or 50 mg/L. A sizable number of foods, such as simple jams, citrus and orange concentrates, starch, sago and fermented vinegar, contains lower levels of sulfites that can still cause reactions. Another problem is e.g. added fruits in yoghurt since the sorbic acid used by some companies for conserving the fruits need not be declared. In case of doubt, only food with the clear inscription "without preservatives" should be considered to be definitely free from additives. The inscription "without added preservatives" merely indicates on the other hand that the producer himself has not added any substances.

Fortunately, many producers currently try to avoid the addition of preservatives. Thus, many sliced breads no longer contain sorbic acid and are instead treated with heat, many salad sauces are currently sold without benzoic acid, and sorbic acid in margarine has mostly been replaced by citric acid. In ice-cream, industry still tends to use natural dyes, but these cause far fewer reactions than azo- and other synthetic dyes.

The detection and avoidance of food additives by patients with pseudoallergies will probably remain a major challenge, now and in the future, since despite international efforts to harmonize the use of food additives, new chemicals whose pseudoallergenic potential is currently unknown, are successively introduced into processed food.

11.2.3
Specific Immunotherapy

IgE-mediated allergies can under certain conditions be treated by specific immunological desensitization, its endpoint being tolerance of the specific allergen. This treatment is time-consuming, potentially dangerous and can therefore only be done by an experienced physician. Desensitization is currently practiced most successfully with highly sensitized bee and wasp allergic patients, particularly when they are in danger because of frequent exposure. Other indications are drug allergies (penicillin, insulin, isoniazide, diphenyl-hydantoine etc.), progesterone allergy and more recently allergies against monoclonal antibodies which are used therapeutically to prevent rejection of transplantated organs. At times, rush desensitization (within 24 hours) may be indicated in patients highly sensitized to penicillin when this antibiotic is the only and most effective drug. Not all allergens are equally suitable for hyposensitization. Monoallergens are generally more effective than antigen mixes.

Hyposensitization against bee and wasp allergies is done with commercially available venom extracts, traditionally on an ambulatory basis. In Europe, the so-called rush hyposensitization is generally used for initiation of treatment. In that case, patients are given 3–4 subcutaneous injections per day while they are hospitalized, starting with 0.2 ml of a 100fold dilution of the lowest titer that is positive on prick testing. After 4–5 days, the undiluted venom is generally tolerated at a full dose, and the patient is thus generally protected from life-threatening reactions. Although this desensitization procedure is well tolerated, with only rare serious reactions (Greineder 1996), it should always be done with an indwelling intravenous catheter and with the patient under constant observation. Maintenance therapy must be done for about three years, in highly sensitized patients possibly even for 5-10 years, with increasing intervals between injections (Keating et al. 1991; Golden et al. 1996).

For other allergens, a similar schedule of desensitization can be employed. Good results are however limited to insect venoms, inhalation allergens and penicillin. In patients who need a full dose of the allergen as rapidly as possible (e.g. for penicillin therapy in streptococcal endocarditis), the endpoint of desensitization can be reached within a day. In this case, increasing doses are given subcutaneously at 15 minute intervals. Once a dose of 800000 IU is tolerated, treatment can be switched to continuous i.v. infusions. Since most patients have allergic symptoms during this entire period (the goal is a "controlled anaphylaxis"), this rapid desensitization can only be done in an intensive care unit, with constant monitoring and readily available resuscitation equipment (Borish et al. 1987). In the future, one can expect suitably tailored peptides or receptor antibodies for improvement of the currently still crude and complex immunotherapy regimens (DeVries 1994).

11.3 Mast Cell-Directed Therapy

This approach is limited to only a few available treatment modalities. Thus, the releasability of mast cell mediators can be reduced pharmacologically, particularly by β-adrenergic agents, calcium blockers like nifedipin or flunarizine or by corticosteroids. The latter also reduce the number of mast cells after local intensive treatment (fluorinated preparations under occlusion). The same effect can also be achieved with PUVA (see treatment of urticaria pigmentosa, Chapter 9). In both situations, the effect of treatment is not persistent.

Corticosteroids as well as PUVA are not suitable for the treatment of chronic urticaria because of their long-term potentially serious adverse effects. Short-term treatment with corticosteroids is, however, highly effective and also justifiable in acute urticaria, particularly when the eliciting agent is apparent and the patient is otherwise healthy (Zuberbier et al. 1996). Because of its low absorption from the gastrointestinal tract, the mast cell stabilizing agent disodium-cromoglycate is of little use in urticaria. In patients with mastocytosis and gastrointestinal symptoms and in patients with genuine food allergies, it is however highly effective in the control of the intestinal symptomatology (Soter et al. 1979; Czarnetzki and Behrendt 1981). The mast cell stabilizing effects, as observed in vitro for some newer non-sedating antihistamines, are however of questionable clinical relevance, probably because the high drug levels necessary for these effects can not be reached in the tissue. Treatment of urticaria with inhibitors of histamine synthesis, e.g. tritoqualin, is according to our own experience of little use in suppressing the symptomatology of whealing reactions.

Patients who suffer from types of urticaria associated with a refractory period can use the latter effectively to control their symptoms. The refractory period is apparently due to an exhaustion of histamine stores within mast cells. Patients can be instructed to regularly expose their skin to stimuli which fail to provoke severe reactions but still keep histamine stores depleted. In the absence of major histamine synthesis, these patients can thus keep their symptomatology at a low level on reexposure. This type of treatment is particularly useful in patients with physical and cholinergic urticaria as well as in patients with contact urticaria.

11.4 Therapy at the Target Organ

11.4.1 Antihistamines

Inhibition or amelioration of symptoms is the most common type of treatment of urticaria (Fig. 11.1). Until antihistamines became available, this type of therapy could only be done with poorly effective means like shake lotions, possibly with menthol added. With the availability of antihistamines since the 1950's, urticarial reactions can almost invariably be effectively suppressed. There is hardly any other disease for which such effective treatment, together with a relatively low adverse effect profile, is available (Simons 1992). Histamine exerts its effects via three different types of receptors:

- *H_1-receptors* which mediate vascular permeability, itching and contraction of the smooth musculature
- *H_2-blockers* which regulate secretion of gastric acid and which are also expressed on subtypes of lymphocytes as well as on basophil leukocytes
- the recently discovered *H_3-receptor* which regulates the synthesis and release of histamine from basophils, as does the H_2 receptor, and which has otherwise been primarily identified in the CNS and at free nerve endings in the periphery.

With few exceptions, practically all symptoms of urticaria are mediated via H_1-receptors. H_1-receptor antagonists are thus of eminent importance in the treatment of urticaria.

The choice of different H_1-antagonists should be guided by clinical aspects as well as by the pharmacological properties of the specific preparation: All H_1-blockers bind competitively and reversibly to specific receptors in the tissue so that prophylactic therapy is most effective. The more recently developed second generation antihistamines differ from older sedating type antihistamines by the absence of, or reduction of effects on the CNS (Fig. 11.2). All H_1-antagonists are well absorbed and reach maximal plasma levels within 1–2 h. The plasma half life varies among different substances, and the biological effect varies even more so since in some preparations, the metabolites are effective as well and may be eliminated more slowly than the parent substance (Table 11.2). The duration of action of H_1-antihistamines of the first generation is relatively short (2–6 h), while second generation antihistamines only reach maximal plasma levels by this time. Astemizole is an exception since its plasma levels increase very slowly, and the pharmacological effects are maintained over many weeks. For this reason, astemizole is not suitable for the treatment of acute urticaria. It can however be used like other H_1-blockers

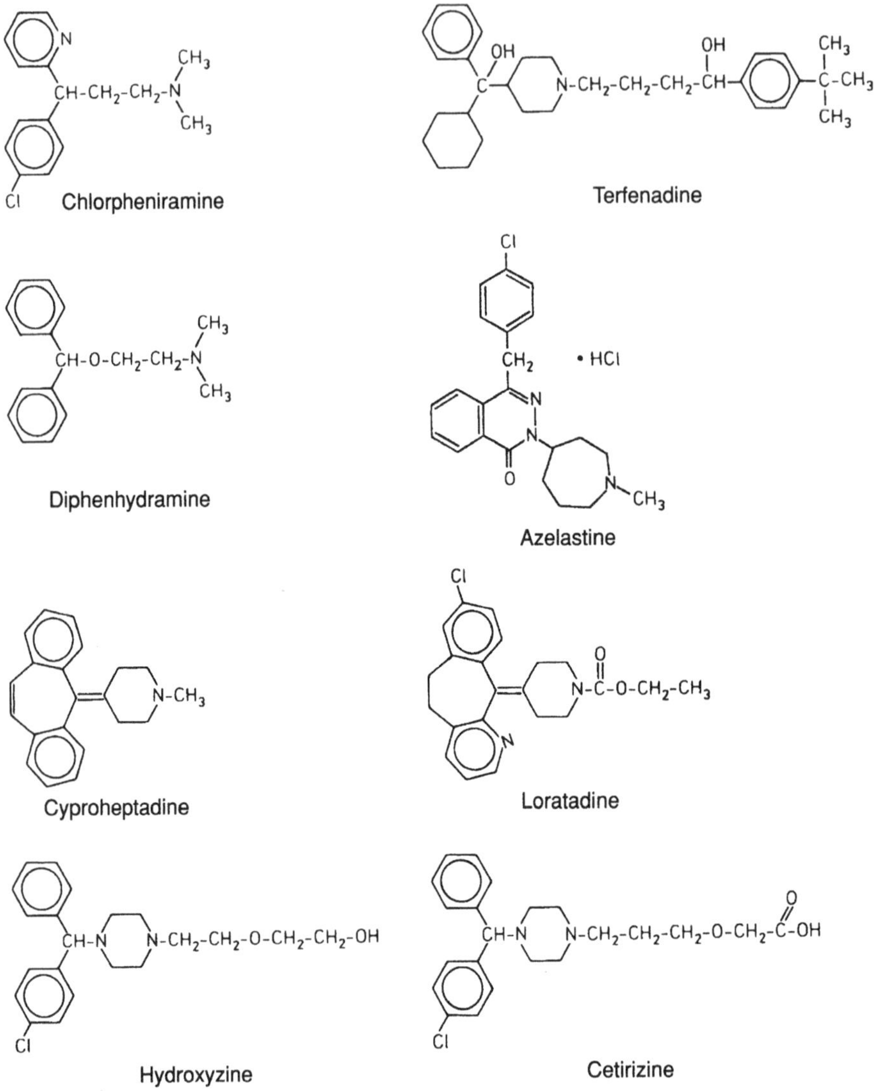

Fig. 11.2. Structure of the most important types of the first (left) and second (right) generation H1-antagonists. Chlorpheniramine belongs to the class of alkylamines, diphenhydramine to the ethanolamines, cyproheptadine to the piperidines and hydroxyzin to the piperazines. Cetirizine is also a piperazine

during maintenance therapy in chronic urticaria, although all diagnostic procedures should be concluded before start of treatment. Tachyphylaxis of the tissue does not occur with antihistamines so that long term therapy does not require an increase of the dose.

Almost all H_1-antagonists are primarily metabolized by the P_{450} system in the liver. Adverse effects like tiredness from first generation antihistamines are

Table 11.2. Pharmacological properties and special aspects of second generation H_1 antagonists. The half maximal elimination time is given for healthy adults. T_{max} = time until reaching maximal plasma levels after oral intake; $t_{1/2}$ = plasma half-life; * for the active loratadine metabolite: 17–24 h; + holds only for the active metabolite of terfenadine; ** first and second pass

Substance	T_{max} [h]	$t_{1/2}$ [h]	Dose [mg/day]	Special aspects
Cetirizine	0.9	7.4	10	Antieosinophilotactic, antineutrophilotactic, inhibition of LTC_4, PGD_2 release
Loratadine	1.0	7.8–11*	10	Inhibition of histamine, LTC_4, PGD_2 release, inhibition of calcium flux, reduction of bradykinin and tame esterase activity
Terfenadine	1.0	17^+	120	Potential cardiotoxicity
Astemizole	3.0	≥228	10	Antiserotinergic, biological effects over many weeks, potential cardiotoxicity,
Ketotifen	2.9	3 + 20**	1–2	Anticholinergic
Azelastine	5.1	22.2	4	Inhibition of histamine, LTC_4 and PAF release, calcium flux, calcium release and formation of oxygen radicals

therefore increased during alcohol intake or treatment with sedatives like diazepam, and plasma levels are increased in older persons and in patients with liver damage. Children metabolize the drugs more rapidly. Cetirizine, the active, non-sedating metabolite of hydroxyzine, is not metabolized in the liver and is largely excreted in the kidney so that levels are increased in patients with renal damage and in older persons. All H_1-antagonists are secreted with breast milk. There are currently no contraindications to treatment of first and second generation H_1-blockers in children, although not all preparations are registered for this age group.

Antihistamines of the H_1 type are the mainstay in the management of urticaria. They may be divided into various pharmacologic groups, which in general have similar properties. Many of these agents are moderately effective in controlling the signs and symptoms of urticaria.

Of the first-generation or classic H_1 antihistamines, a few agents deserve specific mention. Hydroxyzine hydrochloride has been used often as the first-line treatment of urticaria. Part of this popularity may be a result of its multiple properties as an antihistamine, sedative, and antiserotonin agent. Thus, hydroxyzine has been shown to be more effective than other classic antihistamines in inhibiting wheal-and-flare skin reactions, in suppressing histamine-induced pruritus, in dermographism, and in cholinergic urticaria (Monroe 1988). The usual starting dose is 10 to 25 mg four times per day.

When a classic antihistamine fails to be helpful, the dosage should be increased to the highest tolerable and safe level. If a first generation antihistamine is combined with a second generation antihistamine, the first generation antihistamine can be prescribed at night to lessen the potential for sedation.

The usefulness of the first generation antihistamines is sometimes limited by undesirable adverse effects, especially central nervous system effects such as daytime sedation and anticholinergic effects such as dry mouth (Table 11.3). Because of these problems, extensive research has led to the development of a new class of peripherally acting, second generation antihistamines.

When the potency of different newer type antihistamines was compared using the model of histamine wheals on prick testing, cetirizine was noted to be most potent, with a duration of action for 24 hours. Terfenadine (120 mg) was just as effective, but the effect already decreased after 24 hours. Loratadine (10 mg) is less effective in this model, although it is far better than placebo or

Table 11.3. Potential adverse effects of H_1 receptor antagonists

Target organ	Adverse effect
CNS	Sedation, tiredness, sluggishness, problems with coordination, euphoria, insomnia, tremor, nervousness, increased appetite
Eyes	Decreased visual acuity, diplopia
Ears	Tinnitus, dizziness
Muscles	Weakness, muscle twitching
Gastro intestinal tract	Loss of appetite, dryness of mouth, nausea, vomiting, diarrhea, constipation, stomach pains
Immune system	Urticaria, maculopapular rash, photosensitivity (promethazine, tripolidin), contact allergy
Teratogenicity	In animals: piperazine and hydroxyzine in humans: brompheniramine; possible association with retrolental fibrosis
Reproductive system	Problems with erection at high doses

chlorpheniramine (4 mg), a first generation antihistamine (Simons et al. 1990). Review of published clinical studies comparing the efficacy of the newer antihistamines in chronic urticaria shows that in the vast majority of studies, the agents demonstrate statistically equivalent efficacy. Therefore, the histamine-induced wheal and flare test is not a reliable indicator of the comparative clinical efficacy of different antihistamines in the treatment of allergic diseases.

In clinical studies, the potency of hydroxyzine and its non-sedating metabolite cetirizine are comparable. In a recent study comparing cetirizine and azelastine in pruritic dermatoses, cetirizine was however more effective in suppressing whealing, while azelastine was superior in suppressing pruritus (Henz et al. 1997). Cetirizine is not only an H_1-blocker, but it also inhibits the migration of eosinophil and neutrophil granulocytes into the tissue and, like azelastine and loratadine, it inhibits the release of leukotriene C_4. Similar effects have been described for mizolastine (Brostoff et al. 1996). Loratadine has no clear antieosinophilic effects in humans, but it is a potent inhibitor of cytokine-release from mast cells (Lippert et al. 1996). All these substances can thus potentially reduce the associated inflammation in urticarial reactions (Czarnetzki 1986, 1994; Simons 1992, Kenneth and Ellis 1991).

First generation H_1-antihistamines are also used to treat sea sickness, and at higher doses, they act as local antipruritics.

The most serious *undesired adverse effects* of first generation H_1-antagonists (Fig. 11.2) are central sedating effects (Table 11.3). These drugs should therefore be ordered at initially low and then increasing doses so that patients become tolerant to symptoms of tiredness. Additional adverse effects relate to antagonistic actions against serotonin and acetylcholine. Antihistamines generally do not accumulate and can apparently be taken over long periods of time without an increase of adverse effects.

In case of *overdosage* and in children, there can be overexcitation of the CNS, and higher doses can induce epileptic attacks in predisposed patients. There are no specific antidotes. These effects are most likely due to mechanisms other than H_1-blockade. Symptoms of overdosage are overactivity, insomnia, hallucinations, fever, dilatation of the pupils, urinary retention, decreased intestinal peristalsis, drop of blood pressure, tachycardia and cardiac arrhythmias. Death results from central coma and cardiac arrest, in centrally inactive antihistamines (until now only known for astemizole and terfenadin) primarily via cardiovascular effects (drop of blood pressure, cardiac arrest). Because of potentially life threatening cardiac arrhythmias on overdosage with the latter two drugs, these should not be given simultaneously with agents that are also metabolized by the P_{450} system in the liver, such as erythromycin or ketoconazole or with cardiac drugs that prolong the QT interval (Kemp 1992).

Second generation antihistamines (Fig. 11.2) have the major advantage of either not penetrating the blood-brain-barrier or not binding to receptors in the brain. They therefore cause no or only minor tiredness at the recommended dosage. Ketotifen, astemizole as well as the older sedating cyproheptadine increase the patient's appetite and thus can cause weight gain.

In clinical studies of chronic urticaria patients treated with newer, second generation antihistamines (Table 11.1), these drugs have proved statistically superior to placebo and clinically comparable to medium- and high-strength classic antihistamines such as chlorpheniramine and hydroxyzine (Monroe 1988). Clinical studies comparing the second generation antihistamines with each other have generally shown no statistically significant differences among the new agents, with the exception of pruritus versus whealing in a comparison of azelastine versus cetirizine (Henz et al. 1997). Results of several other clinical studies with non-sedating antihistamines can be summarized as follows:

Terfenadine has been shown in clinical studies to be statistically superior to placebo (Cerio and Lessof 1984; Krause and Shuster 1985; Ferguson et al. 1985), equal or superior to clemastine (Fredriksson et al. 1986) and comparable to chlorpheniramine (Grant et al. 1988). A 6-week (optional 12-week) multicenter study involving 158 patients with chronic idiopathic urticaria compared terfenadine, hydroxyzine, and placebo (Monroe et al. 1992). Both terfenadine and hydroxyzine provided significant improvement for all physician and patient evaluations at 6 and 12 weeks of active treatment. Terfenadine and hydroxyzine were not significantly different for any parameter at any visit. The incidence of sedation, however, was four times greater in the hydroxyzine group. Fexofenadine, a metabolite of terfenadine without the cardiovascular side effects, has recently been approved in the United States (1996) and will probably replace terfenadine for use in allergic conditions.

Loratadine has been shown in clinical studies to be statistically superior to placebo (Monroe 1988; Belaich et al. 1990). A 4-week (optional 12-week) multicenter study involving 172 patients with chronic idiopathic urticaria compared loratadine, hydroxyzine, and placebo (Monroe 1991). Both loratadine and hydroxyzine provided significant improvement for all physician and patient evaluations at 1, 4 and 12 weeks of active treatment. Loratadine and hydroxyzine were not significantly different for any evaluation parameter at any visit. The incidence of sedation, however, was significantly greater with hydroxyzine than with either loratadine or placebo, which were comparable.

Cetirizine has been shown in clinical studies to be statistically superior to placebo (Spector and Altman 1987; Juhlin and Arendt 1988). A 4-week multicenter study involving 211 patients with chronic idiopathic urticaria compared cetirizine, hydroxyzine, and placebo (Kalivas et al. 1990). Both cetirizine and hydroxyzine provided significant improvement; they were clinically equivalent in efficacy. In cholinergic urticaria, cetirizine is also highly effective although higher doses may need to be instituted (Zuberbier et al. 1995a).

11.4.2 Further Therapeutic Possibilities

Practicing physicians are well aware of the fact that certain patients with urticaria will not respond to any of the treatments mentioned so far. This holds particularly for patients with urticarial vasculitis and delayed pressure urticaria. Both of these types of urticaria respond to corticosteroids, generally at low daily doses (5–10 mg prednisone daily or q.o.d.). Because of their potential side effects, these drugs are however mostly not suitable for maintenance therapy. The same holds for cyclosporin A (Fradin et al. 1991) and stanozolol (Helfman and Falangen 1995).

Alternatively, combinations of H_1- and H_2-blockers, tricyclic antidepressants, -adrenergic substances, calcium antagonists and inhibitors of inflammatory reactions like dapsone alone or in combination with pentoxifyllin or PUVA may be tried instead. In some patients with a high level of anxiety or depression, the symptoms of urticaria were also more effectively suppressed with a combination of H_1-blockers and benzodiazepines (Hashiro and Yamatidani 1996).

Therapeutic Alternatives in Patients Not Responding to Usual Treatment Modalities and High-Dose H_1-Antihistamines (Czarnetzki 1994; Tharp 1996)

Combination: dapsone and pentoxifyllin
Combination: H_1-blocker and β-sympathomimetic (e.g. terbutaline)
Combination: H_1 and H_2-blocker
Combination: H_1-blocker and psychotropic drugs
Calcium antagonists (fluranizine, nifedipine)
Complement inhibitors (aprotinin, tranexamic acid)
Tricyclic antidepressants (doxepin)
Danazole (stanozolol)
Dapsone
Interferon α
PUVA
Corticosteroids
Cyclosporin A
Chlorquine
Sulfazalazine
Plasmapheresis
Immunoglobulins

In severely affected patients not responding satisfactorily to H_1-antihistamines, a trial with a tricyclic antidepressant may be worthwhile since these agents are known to exert potent in vitro H_1-antihistaminic effects. Doxepin, a heterocyclic variant of amitryptiline, was found to be approximately 700 times more potent than diphenhydramine on a molar basis as an in vitro H_1-inhibitor (Richelson 1979). Doxepin has also been shown to be a potent in vivo inhibitor of histamine-induced wheal reactions in human skin (Sullivan 1982). Some evidence exists that tricyclic antidepressants may also exert H_2-antihistaminic effects. Clinical studies have shown doxepin to be effective in chronic urticaria (Goldsobel et al. 1986; Green et al. 1985; Harto et el. 1985), and cold urticaria (Neittaanmäki et al. 1984). Doxepin has proved statistically superior to placebo and diphenhydramine and clinically comparable to hydroxyzine (unpublished data). In terms of safety, doxepin has a similar sedation and anticholinergic profile to the first-generation, sedating antihistamines.

Human skin blood vessels have been shown to possess H_2-receptors as well as the commonly recognized H_1 receptors (Greaves et al. 1977). H_1-antihistamines alone thus do not block all of the available histamine receptors in the skin. The clinical studies reported to date for combined H_1- and H_2-antihistamines (cimetidine and ranitidine) in treating chronic idiopathic urticaria have however produced mixed results (Cook and Shuster 1983; Harvey et al. 1981; Monroe et al. 1981; Paul and Bodecker 1988). Several studies have shown combined H_1- and H_2-antihistamine therapy to be statistically more effective than H_1-antihistamine therapy alone in patients with dermographism (Matthews et al. 1979; Kaur et al. 1981; Mansfield et al. 1983). The usual dosage of cimetidine is 300 mg four times per day; that of ranitidine is 150 mg two times per day. Finally, one should not use H_2-antihistamines alone because it is necessary to block all histamine receptors (H_1 and H_2).

There are individual positive reports of trials with complement inhibitors (tranexamic acid, aprotinin) and the antiandrogen danazol. In some patients with long-standing, cortisone-dependent chronic urticaria or urticarial vasculitis, we have been able to reduce symptoms or even induce complete remission with a low dose interferon-α treatment (3×3 million I. U./week) (Czarnetzki et al. 1994). Interferon-β was ineffective. Treatment with sulfasalazine (e.g. azulfidine) or the combination of dapsone and pentoxfyllin can be effective in individual patients with steroid-dependent chronic urticaria or urticarial vasculitis (Nürnberg et al. 1994). In a patient with progesterone-induced urticaria, buserelin, a gonadotropin-releasing hormone analogue, induced a complete remission of symptoms (Yee and Cunliffe 1994).

Systemic corticosteroids are highly effective in severe acute urticaria (Zuberbier et al. 1996) and may be indicated in severe serum sickness and pressure urticaria. They have no place as regular therapy in chronic urticaria, although they may occasionally be used temporarily to break the cycle of a resistant case. If successful in such cases, they should be discontinued as soon as possible or at most maintained on an alternate-day basis. Systemic corticosteroids may have a therapeutic role in cases where immune complexes or complement activation is involved in the pathogenesis of urticaria.

11.5 Prophylactic Therapy

Patients with well-documented severe reactions to certain diagnostic agents (X-ray contrast media) or drugs (e.g. histamine liberators during operative procedures, particularly in mastocytosis) can be exposed to these same agents if urgently needed after a prophylactic therapy with corticosteroids and antihistamines. Several protocols for such treatments have so far been examined. These data suggest that H_1-antihistamines alone are sufficient, that the addition of H_2-blockers is generally favorable, and that corticosteroids are not essential. Although urticarial reactions can not always be prevented by this prophylactic treatment, severe life threatening reactions were never observed.

11.6 Emergency Treatment

Every physician must be familiar with the emergency treatment of patients with severe allergic or intolerance reactions. Instructions of the nursing personal must occur at regular intervals, and emergency drugs must be regularly checked for availability and expiration dates.

Emergency Treatment of Patients with Acute Urticaria, Shortness of Breath and Shock (The patient should be placed in shock position in the latter two conditions and resuscitation equipment should be readily available)

1. *Acute urticaria and angioedema*
   a) Removal of the eliciting agent if possible (bee stinger, induction of vomiting, application of a tourniquet, cooling of local reactions with ice (local injections around the lesions with adrenaline 1:10000, maximally 3 ml)
   b) Patient reassurance and instruction to return immediately in case of shortness of breath
   c) Oral treatment with H_1-blockers or prednisone
   d) Shake lotions for local treatment if desired

2. *Shortness of breath*
   a) Procedure as in 1a; additionally 0.3–0.5 ml adrenaline 1:1000 subcutaneously

b) Intravenous fluid (e.g. normal saline)
c) H_1-antihistamines i.v. (e.g. 2–4 mg clemastine)
d) Corticosteroids i.v.: 250 mg prednisolone initially, up to total dose of 2 g/24 h
e) Inhaled β_2-mimetics (e.g. fenoterole); in case of moderate cardiovascular reactions: epinephrine per medihaler or 0.3–0.5 ml adrenaline 1:1000 subcutaneously, repeatedly every 15 minutes
f) Theophylline (e.g. solosin), 1–2 ampules slowly i.v. (in case of bronchospasm)
g) Possibly oxygen via nasal tubing
h) In case of laryngeal edema, adrenaline medihaler
i) In case of severe unresponding laryngeal edema: intubation, tracheotomy (control breathing and pulse)

3. *Anaphylactic shock*
   a) Adrenaline 1:10000, up to 3 ml slowly i.v.
   b) Further therapy as under 2b–d (constantly controlling breathing and pulse).

If urticarial reactions are the only symptoms, the situation is not dangerous. Patients with acute reactions should have the blood pressure checked, and in case of a decrease the patient must be placed flat on the back in shock position, with the subsequent procedures as mentioned above. If after 2 hours of observation there are no symptoms other than urticaria, the patient can be sent home with antihistamines or possibly also corticosteroids. In severe reactions, adrenaline is the most rapidly effective drug. Antihistamines and corticosteroids should be given initially as well, but they need at least one half hour until good clinical effectiveness even after intravenous application.

Infusion of calcium, as is practiced in some countries, is not effective in the treatment of urticaria and acute anaphylactic shock. Calcium is however helpful when the patient hyperventilates and when tetanus can not be otherwise treated effectively (breathing into a bag is generally a more effective and simple therapy).

Literature

Belaich S, Bruttman G, DeGreef H, Lachapelle TM, Paul E, Pedrali P, Tennstedt O (1990) Comparative effects of laratadine and terfenadine in the treatment of chronic idiopathic urticaria. Ann Allergy 64:191–194

Borish L, Tamir R, Rosenwasser LJ (1987) Intravenous desensitization to beta-lactam antibiotics. J Allergy Clin Immunol 80:314–319

Brostoff J, Fitzharris P, Dunmore C, Theron M, Blondin P (1996) Efficacy of mizolastine, a new antihistamine, compared with placebo in the treatment of chronic idiopathic urticaria. Allergy 51:320–325

Cerio R, Lessof MH (1984) Treatment of chronic idiopathic urticaria with terfenadine. Clin Allergy 14:139-141
Cook LJ, Shuster S (1983) Lack of effect of cimetidine in chronic idiopathic urticaria. Acta Dermatol Venereol 63:265-267
Czarnetzki BM, Behrend H (1981) Urticaria pigmentosa: clinical picture and response to oral disodium cromoglycate. Brit J Dermatol 105:563-567
Czarnetzki BM (1986) Urticaria. Springer, Berlin Heidelberg New York Tokyo
Czarnetzki BM, Algermissen B, Jeep S, Haas N, Nürnberg W, Müller K, Kropp J-D (1994) Interferone treatment of patients with chronic urticaria and mastocytosis. J Am Acad Dermatol 30:500-501
Czarnetzki BM (1991) Chronic urticaria. In: Lichtenstein LM, Fauci AS (ed) Current therapy in allergy, immunology and rheumatology. 4th edn. Decker, Toronto, pp 49-52
Czarnetzki BM (1994) Neues zur Diagnostik und Therapie der Urtikaria. Allergologie 17:2-5
DeVries JE (1994) Novel fundamental approaches to intervening in IgE-mediated allergic diseases. J Invest Dermatol 102:141-144
Ferguson J, MacDonald KJS, Kenicer KJA (1985) Terfenadine and placebo compared in the treatment of chronic idiopathic urticaria: a randomized double-blind study. Br J Clin Pharmacol 20:639-641
Fradin MS, Ellis CN, Goldfarb MT, Voorhees JJ (1991) Oral cyclosporin for severe chronic idiopathic urticaria and angioedema. J Am Acad Dermatol 25:1065-1067
Fredriksson T, Herslek T, Hjorth N (1986) Terfenadine in chronic urticaria: a comparison with clemastine and placebo. Cutis 38:128-130
Gibson A, Clancy R (1980) Management of chronic idiopathic urticaria by the identification and exclusion of dietary factors. Clin Allergy 10:699-704
Golden DBK, Kwiterovich KA, Kagey-Sobotka A, Valentine MD, Lichtenstein LM (1996) Discontinuing venom immunotherapy: Outcome after five years. J Allergy Clin Immunol 97:579-587
Goldsobel AB, Rohr AS, Siegel SC, Spector SL, Katz RM, Rachelefsky GS, Drayton G, Indianer L, Peter JB, Barr RJ (1986) Efficacy of doxepin in the treatment of chronic idiopathic urticaria. J Allergy Clin Immunol 78:867-873
Grabbe J, Czarnetzki BM (1992) Akute und chronische Urtikaria. Dt. Med. Wochenschr 117: 1365-1370
Grant JA, Bernstein DI, Buckley CE, Chu T, Fox R, Rocklin R, Schoenwetter W, Spector S, Stafford C, Stroh T, Karpenter K (1988) Double-blind comparison of terfenadine, chlorpheniramine and placebo in the treatment of chronic idiopathic urticaria. J Allergy Clin Immunol 81:574-579
Greaves M, Marks R, Robertson I (1977) Receptors for histamine in human skin blood vessels: a review. Br J Dermatol 97:262-266
Greene SL, Reed CE, Schroeter AL (1985) Double-blind crossover study comparing doxepin with diphenhydramine for the treatment of chronic urticaria. J Am Acad Dermatol 12: 669-675
Greineder DK (1996) Risk management in allergen immunotherapy. J Allergy Clin Immunol 98:330-334
Harto A, Sentagorda E, Ledo A (1985) Doxepin in the treatment of chronic urticaria. Dermatologica 170:90-95
Harvey RP, Wegs J, Schocket AL (1981) A controlled trial of therapy in chronic urticaria. J Allergy Clin Immunol 68:262-266
Hashiro M, Yamatodani Y (1996) A combination therapy of psychotropic drugs and antihistaminics or antiallergics in patients with chronic urticaria. J Dermatol Sci 11: 209-213

Haustein U (1996) Pseudoallergen-free diet in the treatment of chronic urticaria. Acta Derm Venereol (Stockh) 76:498-499

Helfman T, Falanga V (1995) Stanozolol as a novel therapeutic agent in dermatology. J Am Acad Dermatol 32:254-258

Henz BM, Zuberbier T, O'Keefe E, Metzenauer P (1997) Differential effects of new generation H_1-receptor antagonists in pruritic dermatoses. Allergy, submitted

Juhlin L (1981) Recurrent urticaria: clinical investigation of 330 patients. Br J Dermatol 104:369-381

Juhlin L, Arendt C (1988) Treatment of chronic urticaria with cetirizine dihydrochloride, a non-sedating antihistamine. Br J Dermatol 119:67-72

Kalivas J, Breneman D, Tharp M, Bruce S, Bigby M (1990) Urticaria: clinicl efficacy of cetirizine in comparison with hydroxyzine and placebo. J Allergy Clin Immunol 86: 1014-1018

Kaur S, Greaves M, Eftekhari N (1981) Factitious urticaria (dermographism): treatment of cimetidine and chlorpheniramine in a randomized double blind study. Br J Dermatol 104:185-190

Keating MU, Kagey-Sobotka A, Hamilton RG, Yunginger JW (1991) Clinical and immunological follow-up of patients who stop venom immunotherapy. J Allergy Clin Immunol 88:339-348

Kenneth CD, Ellis CN (1991) Pharmacologic therapy for urticaria. J Am Acad Dermatol 25: 176-189

Kemp JP (1992) Antihistamines - is there anything safe to prescribe? Ann Allergy 69: 276-280

Krause L, Shuster S (1983) Mode of action of H1 antihistamines in itch. Br J Dermatol 109 (Suppl 24):30

Lippert U, Krüger-Krasagakes S, Möller A, Kiessling U, Czarnetzki BM (1995) Pharmacological modulation of IL-6 and IL-8 secretion by the H1-antagonist descarboethoxyloratadine and dexamethasone from human mast and basophilic cell lines. Exp Dermatol 4:272-276

Mansfield LE, Smith JA, Nelson HS (1983) Greater inhibition of dermographia with combination of H1 and H2 antagonists. Ann Allergy 50:264-265

Matthews CNA, Boss JM, Warin RP, Storari F (1979) The effect of H1 and H2 histamine antagonists on symptomatic dermographism. Br J Dermatol 101:57-61

Monroe EW, Cohen SH, Kalbfleisch J, Schulz CT (1981) Combined H1 and H2 antihistamine therapy in chronic urticaria. Arch Dermatol 117:404-407

Monroe EW (1988) Chronic urticaria: review of non-sedating H1 antihistamines in treatment. J Am Acad Dermatol 19:842-849

Monroe EW, Fox R, Kalivas J, Katz I, Bernstein D, Honsinger R, Grabier S, Garvin P, Cuss F, Lutsky B (1991) Comparative efficacy and safety of loratadine, hydroxyzine, and placebo in chronic idiopathic urticaria. J Allergy Clin Immunol 87:224

Monroe EW, Bernstein D, Bronsky E, Hanifin J, Prenner B, Schoenwetter W, Spector S, Stafford C, Stroh J, Wanderer A (1992) A doubleblind, randomized, placebo controlled, parallel study comparing the safety and efficacy of ternenadine 60 mg bid to hydroxyzine 25 mg qid administered for 6 to 12 weeks in the treatment of chronic idiopathic urticaria [Abstract]. Clin Res Rep 43:1

Neittaanmäki H, Hyöhänen T, Fräki JE (1984) Comparison of cinnarizine, cyproheptadine, doxepin, and hydroxyzine in treatment of idiopathic cold urticaria: Usefulness of doxepin. J Am Acad Dermatol 11:483-489

Nürnberg W, Grabbe J, Czarnetzki BM (1994) Synergistic effects of combined pentoxifylline and dapsone in leukocytoclastic vasculitis. Lancet 343:49

Paul E, Bodeker RH (1986) Treatment of chronic urticaria with terfenadine and ranitidine: a randomized doubleblind study in 45 patients. Eur J Clin Pharm 31:277-280

Richelson E (1979) Tricyclic antidepressants and histamine H1 receptors. Mayo Clin Proc 54:669-674

Rudzki E, Czubalski K, Grzywa Z (1980) Detection of urticaria with food additives intolerance by means of diet. Dermatologica 161:57-62

Simons FR, McMiilan JL, Simons KJ (1990) A double-blind, single-dose crossover comparison of cetirizine, terfenadine, loratadine, astemizole, and chlorpheniramine versus placebo, suppression effects on histamine-induced wheals and flared during 24 hours in normal subjects. A Allergy Clin Immunol 86:540-547

Simons FER (1992) The antiallergic effects of antihistamines (H_1-receptor antagonists). J Allergy Clin Immunol 90:705-715

Soter NA, Austen KF, Wasserman SI (1979) Oral sodium cromoglycate in the treatment of systemic mastocytosis. N Engl J Med 301:465-469

Spector SL, Altman R (1987) Cetirizine, a novel antihistamine. Am J Rhinol 1:147-149

Sullivan T (1982) Pharmacologic modulation of the whealing response to histamine in human skin: identification of doxepin as a potent in vivo inhibitor. J Allergy Clin Immunol 69:260-267

Tharp MD (1996) Chronic urticaria: pathophysiology and treatment approaches. J Allergy Clin Immunol 98:S325-S330

Yee KC, Cunliffe WJ (1994) Progesterone-induced urticaria- response to buserelin. Br J Dermatol 130:121-123

Zuberbier T, Aberer W, Burtin M, Rihoux J-P, Czarnetzki BM (1995a) Efficacy of cetirizine in cholinergic urticaria. Acta Derm Venereol (Stockh) 75:147-149

Zuberbier T, Chantraine-Heß S, Czarnetzki BM (1995b) The role of food intolerance in chronic urticaria - a prospective study. Acta Derm Venereol (Stockh) 75:484-487

Zuberbier T, Iffländer J, Semmler C, Czarnetzki BM (1996) Acute urticaria - clinical aspects and therapeutic responsiveness. Acta Derm Venereol (Stockh) 76:295-297

Appendix A

Urticaria Questionnaire

Name: Department ....
Birth date:
Current date:

Dear Patient,

You have consulted your physician because of chronic urticaria which manifests itself typically by recurring bouts of whealing and/or swelling of the skin. Wheals or urticae are itching elevations or bumps of the skin which vary in size from tiny to large and which disappear after a brief period of time. The condition may also be associated with deep and extensive swellings on any site of the skin, particularly on the eye-lids and the lips. Urticaria may be due to many causes. Their identification requires frequently the qualities of a detective by you and your physician alike. Therefore please take your time in answering this questionnaire as exactly as possible. Do not omit any questions. In most cases, you need to only mark the correct answer. If you are not able to answer a question or if you don't understand it, please write "unclear" on the margin or mark the appropriate box. Your doctor can evaluate the questionnaire more easily if you use a red pen.

Thank you for your cooperation.

1. How long do you suffer from urticaria?

   Since......................................

2. What kind of symptoms do you have?

   ❑ superficial wheals only
   ❑ deep swellings only
   ❑ wheals as well as deep swellings

3. How frequently do you observe superficial wheals?

   ❑ daily
   ❑ several times weekly
   ❑ several times per month
   ❑ more rarely, namely:

4. How frequently do you observe deep, large swellings (angioedema)?

   ❑ daily
   ❑ several times weekly
   ❑ several times per month
   ❑ more rarely, namely:

5. How long do your wheals persist before disappearing?

   ❑ less than 1 hour
   ❑ up to 24 hours
   ❑ longer than 24 hours

6. How long do the deep swellings persist?

   ❑ up to 24 hours
   ❑ up to 72 hours
   ❑ longer than 72 hours

7. How big are the wheals?

   ❑ pin size to pea size
   ❑ larger, namely as big as:

8. Do your wheals preferentially appear at certain sites of the body?

   ❑ no
   ❑ yes, particularly at the following sites:
   ❑ yes, exclusively at the following sites:

9. At which body sites do the deep swellings (angioedemas) appear?

   ❑ on the eye-lids
   ❑ on the lips
   ❑ at other places, namely:

	Yes	Unclear	No
10. Have you ever experienced swellings of the tongue, the palate, the throat? If yes, where exactly:	❑	❑	❑
11. Did the swelling of your neck or throat lead to shortness of breath?	❑	❑	❑

12. At which time of the day do your wheals occur mostly?
    - ❑ in the morning
    - ❑ at noon
    - ❑ in the afternoon
    - ❑ in the evening
    - ❑ at night

	Yes	Un-clear	No
13. Do you sometimes wake up at night because of whealing?	❑	❑	❑
14. Do the wheals leave blue/brownish spots or red dots after they disappear for a few days?	❑	❑	❑
15. Do you notice running of the nose or tearing of the eyes during whealing reactions?	❑	❑	❑
16. Have you ever noticed asthmatic complaints or shortness of breath during whealing reactions?	❑	❑	❑
17. Have you ever noticed the following other symptoms during whealing attacks?			
• joint pains	❑	❑	❑
• swelling at the joints	❑	❑	❑
• abdominal pain	❑	❑	❑
• gastric pain, heart burns	❑	❑	❑
• nausea, vomiting	❑	❑	❑
• diarrhea	❑	❑	❑
• fever	❑	❑	❑
• inflammation of the eyes	❑	❑	❑
• swelling of the lymph nodes	❑	❑	❑
• other symptoms; if yes which ones:	❑	❑	❑
18. Did you or a member of your family ever notice whealing reactions or swellings before?	❑	❑	❑
If yes, who?			
19. Did any member of your family ever suffer from the following diseases?			
• infantile eczema (cradle cap)	❑	❑	❑
• itching eczemas in the arm pits or the back of the knees (atopic eczema)	❑	❑	❑
• hay fever, stuffed nose, attacks of sneezing	❑	❑	❑
• allergic asthma	❑	❑	❑
If yes, who?			

	Now	Formerly	Unclear	No
20. Are you currently suffering or did you ever suffer from any of the following diseases?				
• infantile eczema	❏	❏	❏	❏
• itching eczemas in the arm pits or the back of the knees (atopic eczema)	❏	❏	❏	❏
• hay fever, stuffed nose, attacks of sneezing	❏	❏	❏	❏
• allergic asthma	❏	❏	❏	❏
• liver disease (hepatitis)	❏	❏	❏	❏
• diseases of the kidneys	❏	❏	❏	❏
• diseases of the thyroid gland	❏	❏	❏	❏
• rheumatic diseases, e.g. primary chronic polyarthritis	❏	❏	❏	❏
• inflammation of the teeth or the gums	❏	❏	❏	❏
• inflammation of the ear, nose and throat region (e.g. tonsilitis, sinusitis)	❏	❏	❏	❏
• stomach pain, heart burns	❏	❏	❏	❏
• malignant diseases (if yes, which ones?)	❏	❏	❏	❏

	Yes	Unclear	No
21. Did you suffer from any other diseases that are not mentioned?	❏	❏	❏
If yes, which ones:			
22. Can you remember special events or acute illnesses when your urticaria started?	❏	❏	❏
23. Did you ever notice an association between redness and whealing and the following situations?			
• or contact with cold (cold water, cold weather, cold wind, cold objects, cold food)	❏	❏	❏
• or contact with warmth (warm water, warm objects, warm food)	❏	❏	❏
• overheating of the body (e.g. during physical exercise, sports, sweating, hot shower fever, stress)	❏	❏	❏
• on contact with water	❏	❏	❏
• on exposure to sun (also artificial UV-radiation)	❏	❏	❏
24. Did you ever notice whealing several minutes after scratching or rubbing you skin?	❏	❏	❏
25. Did you ever notice swellings on parts of the body that have been exposed to pressure several hours before (e.g. swelling of the soles after long walking, of the buttocks after prolonged sitting or bicycling)?	❏	❏	❏
26. Did you ever take drugs against urticaria?	❏	❏	❏
If yes, which ones and how frequently:			

	Yes	Un-clear	No
27. Do you regularly take other drugs?	❑	❑	❑
If yes, which ones and how frequently:			
28. Do you take at times the following medications?			
• pain medication (such as aspirin)	❑	❑	❑
• tablets against flu	❑	❑	❑
• antirheumatics	❑	❑	❑
• cough medications	❑	❑	❑
• laxatives	❑	❑	❑
• sleeping pills	❑	❑	❑
• hormones	❑	❑	❑
• vitamins	❑	❑	❑
• antibiotics, particularly penicillin	❑	❑	❑
• homcopathic drugs	❑	❑	❑
• other drugs	❑	❑	❑
If yes, which ones and how frequently:			
29. Do you regularly or occasionally receive injections or infusions (e.g. insulin, vitamin B, shots for hyposensitisation, blood transfusions)?	❑	❑	❑
If yes, which ones and how frequently:			
30. Did you ever notice the development of wheals and swellings after taking tablets (e.g. penicillin or aspirin), after an injection or an infusion?	❑	❑	❑
If yes, specify:			
31. Did you ever notice other problems after having a tablet, an injection or an infusion?	❑	❑	❑
If yes, which ones and what kind of symptoms did you have?			
32. Did you ever notice wheals or swellings after an examination with radio contrast media?	❑	❑	❑
33. Did you ever notice wheals or swellings after vaccinations, e.g. against tetanus?	❑	❑	❑
34. Did you ever notice any of the following signs after eating certain foods (e.g. fish, crustaceans, milk, nuts, tomatoes, chocolate, spices, cheese, strawberries, apples, conserved food)	❑	❑	❑
• tingling and a pelty feeling of the tongue			
• swelling of the tongue or the lips			
• other swellings or wheals			
If yes, after which food?			

	Yes	Un-clear	No
35. Did you ever notice wheals or swellings after drinking certain beverages (e.g. beer, wine, other types of alcohol, chinin containing refreshing beverages like lemonade) If yes, after which ones?	❑	❑	❑
36. Did you ever notice wheals or swellings after eating foods or beverages which contained preservatives (e.g. benzoic acid, sorbic acid)? If yes, after which ones?	❑	❑	❑
37. Do you have an aversion against certain foods? If yes, against which ones?	❑	❑	❑
38. Do you use artificial sweeteners instead of sugar?	❑	❑	❑
39. Do you smoke? If yes, what type, which brand and how many?	❑	❑	❑
40. Did you ever notice that touching the skin with the following substances caused redness or swelling?			
• foods (meat, fish, potatoes, herbs, salad, egg, flour, fruit, vegetables, beverages)	❑	❑	❑
• chemicals, objects at work	❑	❑	❑
• cremes, lotions	❑	❑	❑
• animals	❑	❑	❑
• plants	❑	❑	❑
• wood	❑	❑	❑
• textiles	❑	❑	❑
• drugs	❑	❑	❑
• cosmetics, perfumes	❑	❑	❑
• water	❑	❑	❑
41. What is your profession?			
42. What kind of hobbies do you have?			
43. Are you exposed to vapors or dust during work or hobbies? If yes, which ones:	❑	❑	❑
44. Does your urticaria improve or disappear during vacations?	❑	❑	❑
45. Do you have metallic objects (e.g. a pacemaker, artificial joints, metallic screws, dental implants) or other types of implants in your body? If yes, which ones:	❑	❑	❑

	Yes	Un-clear	No
46. Have you noticed wheals or swellings after insect stings?	❑	❑	❑
If yes, which insects:			
47. Did you ever notice wheals during or shortly after intercourse?	❑	❑	❑

Women only

48. Have you noticed the preferential appearance of wheals or swellings at certain times of the menstrual cycle?	❑	❑	❑
If yes, when?			
49. Do you take contraceptives or other hormones?	❑	❑	❑
If yes, which type and since when: If yes, are your wheals and swellings less intense on days when you don't take these preparations:			

Appendix B

Urticaria Diary

Date	Day	Wheals*	Itching*	Remarks
	1			
	2			
	3			
	4			
	5			
	6			
	7			
	8			
	9			
	10			
	11			
	12			
	13			
	14			
	15			
	16			
	17			
	18			
	19			
	20			
	21			
	22			
	23			
	24			
	25			
	26			
	27			
	28			
	29			
	30			

* 0 = none, 1 = mild, 2 = moderate, 3 = severe, please use this score to express disease severity, if you wish to make additional remarks, please use a separate sheet of paper.

Appendix C

Test Protocol: Physical Urticaria

Physical provocation test for urticaria patients

(please mark positive reactions)

Patient identification

Name:	*Last intake of*	*Date/time of day*
	a) Antihistamines	........./.................
Birth date:	*type:*	
	b) Other medications	
	potentially influencing wheals:	

1. Dermographic urticaria

Date/time of day
........./.................

Device for testing:
body region tested: upper back

Result

5 min			2 h		
W	E	Pr	W	E	Pr

Special types of reactions:
e.g. cholinergic dermographism

2. Pressure urticaria

Date/time of day
........./.................

Body site:

Result

Weight	Area	Duration	Immediate W	Immediate E	Immediate Pr	2 h W	2 h E	2 h Pr	4 h W	4 h E	4 h Pr	8 h W	8 h E	8 h Pr
900 g	10 min													
900 g	20 min													
1800 g	10 min													
1800 g	20 min													
...... g	...... min													
Special remarks:														

3. Heat urticaria

Date/time of day
........./..................

Bath
- Arm
- Whole body

37–41C, 3–10 min (increase if negative)

Result

°C	Duration of application		Immediate			2 h			or.........h		
			W	E	Pr	W	E	Pr	W	E	Pr

Special observations

4. Cold urticaria

Date/time of day
........./..................

Test site:

Result

Type of test	Duration of application	Immediate			After 10 min			2 h			24 h		
		W	E	Pr	W	E	Pr	W	E	Pr	W	E	Pr
Ice cube (beaker with ice water)	3–5 min												
	......min												
Arm bath ......°C	5-10 min												
	......min												
Cold air, 4°C until shivering													
	......min												

Reflex whealing?
Other special observations?

5. Solar urticaria

Date/time of day
........./..................

Test site: back, increasing doses

Result

	Up to 2 h*			24 h			48 h		
	W	E	Pr	W	E	Pr	W	E	Pr
UVA									
UVB									
Visible light									

Special observations?

* Reading times, see Chapters 5.6

6. Cholinergic urticaria

Date/time of day

........./.................

Physical exercise in warm environment or warm bath, check body temperature (> 0.5 °C) rise required for valid test

Result

type of test	W	E	Pr
exercise			
warm bath			

body temperature

before test °C

after test °C

Special observations:

Diagnosis:

Test conducted by:

Responsible physician:

W = wheal E = erythema Pr = pruritus

Appendix D 1

Low Pseudoallergen Diet

Strictly forbidden:
All food containing preservatives, dyes or antioxidants; all industrially processed food should be regarded with suspicion (modified from: Zuberbier T, Czarnetzki BM. Nahrungsmittelunverträglichkeit (II). Hautarzt 1993;44:57–62)

	Allowed	Forbidden
Basic food	Preservative-free bread, potatoes, rice, unprocessed cereals, flour (not self-raising!) rice cakes, durum wheat pasta (without egg)	All others (e.g. pasta with eggs, cake, biscuits, potato chips, crisps)
Fats	Butter, cold pressed plant oils	All others (e.g. margarine, mayonnaise)
Milk products	Fresh milk, cream without stabilizers, white cheese, fromage frais, mild Gouda in small amounts	All others
Food from animals	Fresh meat without seasoning	All others including eggs, sea-food, smoked meat
Vegetables	All except those listed as forbidden (e.g. lettuce, carrots, zucchini, cabbage, broccoli, aspargus)	Artichokes, peas, mushrooms, spinach, rhubarb, tomatoes and tomato products, olives, sweet peppers
Fruit	None	All including dried fruits or fruit juices
Herbs, spices	Salt, sugar, chives, onions	All others including garlic and herbs
Sweets	None	All including chewing gum
Beverages	Milk, mineral water, coffee, black tea	All others including beer, wine, spirits and herbal teas
Spreadings	Honey	All others

Appendix D 2

Expansion of the Low Pseudoallergen Diet After Freedom of Symptoms Has Been Obtained

Add only 1 (!!) food item every 3 days!
Additive effects should be taken into account!

Basic food	No change
Fats	No change
Milk products	Buttermilk other mild cheeses
Animal food	Roast beef pollack, plaice, trout eggs
Vegetables	No change
Fruit	Banana, pear, watermelon
Herbs, spices	Fresh herbs (e. g. basil, parseley)
Sweets	None
Beverages	Buttermilk, peppermint or camomille tea pear juice, juice of permitted vegetables (no seasoning except salt permitted)
Spreadings	Treacle

Appendix E

Low Pseudoallergen Diet – Suggestions for Recipes

I. Ehlers

Baked beetroot
(1 person)

Ingredients:

1	Large raw beetroot
200 g	Potatoes
1	Onion
1–2 tbsp	Olive oil
	Salt

Chop the beetroot and the potatoes. Finely dice the onion. Turn into an ovenproof dish. Spoon over oil and bake covered in the oven at 200 °C for 30–40 minutes, until beetroot is tender. Adjust salt to taste.

Beetroot with yoghurt dressing
(1 person)

Ingredients:

1	Large raw beetroot
150 g	Yoghurt
2 tbsp	Chopped chives
	Salt

Wrap the beetroot in aluminium foil and bake in the oven for 40–50 minutes. Meanwhile mix yoghurt and chives and season with salt.
Goes well with jacket or baked potatoes.

Beetroot and carrot salat
(1 person)

Ingredients:

1	Small raw beetroot
1	Large carrot
1	Small onion
1 tbsp	Olive oil

Coarsely grate the beetroot and the carrot. Finely dice the onion. Combine all ingredients in a mixing bowl. Toss well. Cover and chill until used.

Cucumber salad with yoghurt and chives dressing
(1 person)

Ingredients:

200 g	Cucumber
100 g	Yoghurt
1 tsp	Honey
2 tbsp	Chives
	Salt

Combine the yoghurt, the honey and the chives in a mixing bowl. Adjust salt to taste. Slice cucumber and toss in the dressing. Cover and chill until required.

Jacket potatoes with fromage frais
(1 person)

Ingredients:

300 g	Potatoes
150 g	Fromage frais
100 g	Yoghurt
1	Small onion
2 tbsp	Chopped chives
	salt

Steam the potatoes for about 25 minutes until just tender. Meanwhile finely dice the onion and combine with remaining ingredients in a mixing bowl. Adjust salt to taste.

Baked potatoes in a bed of salt
(1 person)

Ingredients:

300 g	Potatoes
1–2 tbsp	Olive oil
	Coarse salt

Turn coarse salt in an ovenproof dish. Place the potatoes on top of the salt bed and spoon over the oil. Bake in the oven at 200 °C for 30–40 minutes until the potatoes are tender. Goes well with any kind of salad.

Fried potatoes
(1 person)

Ingredients:

300 g	Cooked potatoes
1	Large onion
2 tbsp	Butter or olive oil
	Salt

Slice the cooked potatoes and dice the onion. Melt butter in a frying pan and sauté onions until they are transparent. Add potatoes and fry until they are golden. Adjust salt to taste. Goes well with any kind of salad.

Mashed potatoes
(1 person)

Ingredients:

300 g	Potatoes
1 tbsp	Butter
100 ml	Milk
1 tbsp	Salt

Steam the potatoes for about 25 minutes until just tender. Add butter and milk and mash well. Adjust salt to taste. Goes well with any kind of salad.

Steak with chives butter
(1 person)

Ingredients:

150 g	Steak
1	Large onion
1tbsp	Olive oil
1tbsp	Butter
1tbsp	Chopped chives
1 tsp	Finely diced onion
	salt

Salt the steak mildly. Slice the onion into rings and sauté them in olive oil until they are transparent. Add the steak and fry it from both sides to taste. Meanwhile mix the remaining ingredients and adjust salt to taste.
Goes well with potato dishes and salad.

Burger
(1 person)

Ingredients:

60 g	Minced beef
1 tbsp	Fromage frais
1	Small onion
1 tbsp	Salt
	Olive oil

Dice the onion finely. Combine the minced beef, the fromage frais, the onion and salt to taste in a mixing bowl and toss well. Form a burger and fry it in olive oil.
Place into a bread roll with cucumber, lettuce and cheese if desired.

Stuffed zucchini
(1 person)

Ingredients:

60 g	Minced beef
1 tbsp	Fromage frais
	Small onion
1	Salt
1	Small zucchini
1 tsp	Olive oil

Dice the onion finely. Combine the minced beef, the fromage frais, the onion and salt to taste in a mixing bowl and toss well.
Cut the zucchini in half lengthways and scoop out the flesh leaving a 1 cm "wall". Sprinkle with salt. Place the "shells" into a greased ovenproof dish and stuff with the meat mixture. Bake in the oven at 200 °C for 20–30 minutes until the zucchini is just tender.

Baked zucchini
(1 person)

Ingredients:

1	Small zucchini
1	Small onion
1–2 tbsp	Olive oil
	Salt
50 g	Mild gouda

Slice the zucchini and dice the onion. Place into a greased ovenproof dish and spoon out olive oil. Sprinkle with cheese and bake in the oven at 200 °C for about 30 minutes.
This recipe can be easily done with other vegetables such as broccoli or aubergines, too.

Potato soup
(1 person)

Ingredients:

200 g	Potatoes
150 g	Carrots
1	Small onion
1 tbsp	Butter
	Salt
1 tbsp	Chopped chives

Chop the potatoes and the carrots and finely dice the onion. Melt butter in a saucepan and sauté onions until they are transparent. Add potatoes, carrots and 150 - 200 ml water and bring to boil. Reduce the heat, cover and simmer until the vegetables are just tender. Adjust salt to taste and sprinkle with chives.

Carrot soup
(1 person)

Ingredients:

300 g	Carrots
1 tsp	Honey
100 ml	Cream
	Salt

Chop the carrots and bring to boil in 100 - 150 ml water. Reduce heat, cover and simmer for about 15 minutes until they are just tender. Blend in a liquidizer goblet and add the honey and the cream. Adjust salt to taste.

Millet with carrots and zucchini
(1 person)

Ingredients:

50 g	Millet
150 g	Carrots
100 g	Zucchini
1 tbsp	Butter
	Salt
50 ml	Cream

Wash the millet and bring to boil in 100 - 150 ml water. Reduce heat, cover and simmer for 20 - 30 minutes. Meanwhile slice the vegetables. Melt the butter in a frying pan, add vegetables and sauté them. Stir in the cream and adjust salt to taste. Drain the millet and serve vegetables on a bed of millet.

Vegetable rice
(1 person)

Ingredients:

50 g	Rice
150 g	Broccoli
150 g	Carrots
150 g	Cauliflower
1 tbsp	Butter
	Salt

Wash the rice and bring to boil in 100 - 150 ml water. Reduce heat, cover and simmer for 20-30 minutes. Meanwhile chop broccoli and cauliflower and slice carrots. Melt the butter in a frying pan, add vegetables and sauté them. Adjust salt to taste. Drain the rice and add to the vegetables.

Subject Index

FSC
www.fsc.org
MIX
Papier | Fördert gute Waldnutzung
FSC® C083411

Kolibri 360 GmbH
Ferdinand-Jühlke-Straße 7
99095 Erfurt, Deutschland
produktsicherheit@kolibri360.de